PRACTICAL MATHEMATICS
IN ALLIED HEALTH

PRACTICAL MATHEMATICS IN ALLIED HEALTH

A Textbook for the Medical Disciplines

Marian Waterhouse,
RN, CRNA, BS Nursing Ed, MEd
Colonel, US Army, Retired
Former Director, US Army Program of Instruction
in Anesthesiology for Army Nurse Corps Officers

Urban & Schwarzenberg • Baltimore-Munich 1979

Urban & Schwarzenberg, Inc.
7 E. Redwood Street
Baltimore, Maryland 21202
U.S.A.

Urban & Schwarzenberg
Pettenkoferstrasse 18
D-8000 München 2
GERMANY

Library of Congress Cataloging in Publication Data

Waterhouse, Marian.
    Practical mathematics in allied health.

    Bibliography: p.
    Includes index.
    1. Medicine—Mathematics.   I.   Title.
    R853.M3W37   610'.1'51   79-15317

ISBN 0-8067-2121-9   (Baltimore)
ISBN 3-541-72121-9   (München)

Printed in the United States of America

LK 6-8-82

CONTENTS

APPENDIX   A BRIEF REVIEW OF FRACTIONS AND DECIMALS . 221

Preface

The metric mathematics of the pharmacological and biological sciences has been a source of fear and frustration to a majority of the students in the health sciences. This mathematics text book is written as a result of witnessing this sort of fear as it was experienced by nurse anesthetists, operating room nurses, nurse practitioners, nurse educators, and oral surgery and dental residents who were my students in pharmacology and biochemistry during the past 25 years. Their quick and easy mastery of the metric mathematics involved, taught with a "common sense, no formula" approach, was gratifying. The frequent comment from students who wished that they had been taught with this approach when they were undergraduate students, stimulated the writing of this text.

Section I makes a direct comparison of our metric monetary system with the metric measurement of drugs and solutions. Section II deals with the mathematics of biochemistry, and involves an intensive study of the math of equivalent weights, osmotic pressure, osmolality of solutions, and the pH concept. Section III includes a very simple discussion of statistical analysis. Calculations are kept at an absolute minimum, and emphasis is placed on the interpretation of such statistical data as is found in professional literature. A brief review of the mathematics of fractions and decimals is in the appendix. Problems designed to offer practice in the techniques discussed in the text are presented at the end of each section.

I am indebted to countless former students and colleagues for their interest and encouragement before and during the development of this book. For the editing of the manuscript, I owe a debt of gratitude to my mother. In particular I would like to thank Charles C. Alling, DDS, MS, Professor and Chairman, Department of Oral Surgery, University of Alabama School of Dentistry, Birmingham, Alabama, for his help and encouragement, and for the suggestion that I include the section on statistical analysis. To Jennifer Baker many thanks for her excellent illustrations. Finally, I extend my appreciation to the staff of Urban and Schwarzenberg for its helpful and friendly cooperation in the publication of this textbook.

Marian Waterhouse
San Diego, California

Dedicated to all my students

PRACTICAL MATHEMATICS
IN ALLIED HEALTH

SECTION ONE

USE OF
THE METRIC
SYSTEM
IN MONEY AND
DRUGS

Chapter 1
MONEY
AND
THE METRIC SYSTEM

Counting money in most Western countries, including the United States, is not difficult because it is organized in the *metric system*. The metric system is a *decimal system* of weights and measures based on the meter as a unit of length, and the kilogram as a unit of mass or weight. Derived units include the liter for liquid volume. Thus, the United States money system is a *decimal* system, using the dollar as the basic monetary unit. Similarly, measurement of drugs and solutions in science and medicine is predominantly in the metric, or decimal, system. For this reason, anyone who can count money should be able to figure drug problems with relative ease.

Before discussing drugs, some examples of money problems will be presented.

1. Assume that ten dollars is a sum of money due to be paid. "Ten dollars" can be written in the following ways:
   a. $10 is common.
   b. $10.00 is also common, and shows a decimal that indicates no cents.
   c. 1,000 cents is another way to express ten dollars, but is uncommon.
   d. 1000.00 cents, or 1000.000000¢ would also be correct, but is a silly way to express ten dollars, because the extra zeros serve no purpose and make the expression cumbersome.
2. Suppose that all of the ten-dollar debt has been paid. The transaction can be expressed as follows:
   a. The *entire* amount has been paid, not just part, or a fraction of it. The total amount of the debt has been paid in full.
   b. The *whole* amount has been paid. The whole contains *all* of the component parts or elements of a thing. The whole is a

3

complete entity or system, or a complete unit. In this example, "all," or the "whole" amount of the debt has been paid. That is, $10.00 is a whole unit (or number) because it is the complete or total amount of the debt, not just part of it (See Appendix). It can be said that "all" or "1" of what was owed has been paid when "1" represents the total amount.

Early in the math game it must be learned that every answer in mathematical computations must make *sense*, or it is undoubtedly wrong. Answers should constantly be tested with the question, "Does the answer make *sense*?" Examples of ways to test answers will be presented throughout this chapter.

3. Assume that only five dollars of the ten-dollar debt has been paid. This transaction can be expressed as follows:
    a. cents   500¢
    b. fraction   1/2
    c. decimal   .5
    d. percent   50%
    e. ratio   1:2
    These five equivalents are merely different ways of saying the same thing. Each of them is explained to prove that it is, in fact, equivalent to the others.

FRACTIONS

A fraction is a part of a whole (See Appendix). In the problem above, it is stated that $5 has been paid, and that this is 1/2 of the $10 debt. Mathematically, this fact can be written:

$$\$5 = 1/2 \times \$10.$$

How can this be proved?
Everyone knows that 1/2 of $10 is $5. But if the figures were more complicated, the problem would have to be calculated mathematically to ensure a correct answer. Since $5 is a part of $10, it is written as a fraction, thus:

$\dfrac{\$5}{\$10}$, a fraction, which is reduced to 1/2 (See Appendix).

Now it can be written:

$1/2 \times \$10 = \$5$ (See Appendix for multiplication of fractions).

$1/2 \times \$10.00 = \$5.00$

$1/2 \times 1,000¢ = 500¢$

(If the illustrations to this point do not make sense, the Appendix, and/or elementary texts that discuss and drill in the use of fractions should be reviewed.)

Summary

Two equivalent ways to express the payment of $5 as part of a $10 debt are:

500¢	1/2

DECIMALS

It is stated above that the $5 paid is .5 of the $10 debt. The decimal .5 is more correctly termed a "decimal fraction" (See Appendix). A decimal fraction is a fraction whose denominator is 10, or any power of 10, i.e., 100, 1,000, 10,000, and so forth. The denominator, however, is not written as it is in a common fraction. It is signified by the way the number to the right of the decimal point is written.

In this example, ".5" is verbalized as "five-tenths". The number 5 is immediately to the right of the decimal point, so it is in the tenths column (See Appendix). The denominator of this fraction is therefore 10, and the fraction can be written as .5 or 5/10, which can easily be reduced to the fraction 1/2.

The fraction 1/2 can be changed to a decimal by dividing the numerator by the denominator.

$$1 \div 2 = .5 \qquad \text{(See Appendix)}.$$

Therefore

$$\begin{array}{r} \$10.00 \\ \times \quad .5 \\ \hline \$5.000 \end{array} \qquad \text{OR} \qquad \begin{array}{r} 1,000¢ \\ \times \quad .5 \\ \hline 500.0¢ \end{array}$$

Summary

Three equivalent ways to express the payment of $5 as part of a $10 debt are:

500¢	1/2	.5

PERCENTAGES

It is stated that the $5 paid is 50% of the $10 debt. Percent means "per *hundred*," and is a symbol used to express quantity with relation to a whole. In other words, 100% is the *whole*, or the entire quantity. In this problem, $10 is 100% of the debt, or the whole of it. To say it another way, percent means "divided by 100." A % number is a fraction whose numerator is verbalized, and whose denominator is assumed, or understood, to be 100.

100% means 100/100 (or 100 ÷ 100), which equals 1, or 1.00.

50% means 50/100, which equals 5/10, or .5, or 1/2.

Percent can be calculated by multiplying a decimal equivalent of a fraction by 100/100, and substituting the % sign for the denominator. It is proved above that .5 of the $10 debt has been paid. Therefore

the % paid = .5 × 100/100 = 50/100 or 50%. (The % sign means that the denominator 100 is assumed: 50% = 50/100.)

Percentages as They Are Related to Decimal Fractions

It is proved above that .5 = 50%. From the statement that $5 is 50% of $10, the decimal equivalent of 50% can quickly be calculated:

1.   A decimal point is put immediately before the % sign, thus:

50.%.

(If there is a decimal point already in the %, it is left where it is. Example: 1.5%)
2.   Since 50.% means 50./100, the decimal equivalent will be:

50. ÷ 100 = .5

The decimal point is moved two places to the left. 50 can be divided by 100 by long division:

$$100 \overline{)50.0} \quad .5$$

Summary

Four equivalent ways to express the payment of $5 as part of a $10 debt are:

500¢	1/2	.5	50%

Do the figures make *sense*?

Recognizing Errors

It is proved above that .5 = 50% = 1/2. Suppose an error were made when calculating the percentage equivalent of the decimal fraction .5, and the decimal point were moved two places in the wrong direction.

This answer would not make *sense*:

> .5 = .005%
>
> WRONG!!!

Since % means hundredths:

.005% means .005/100;

.005 ÷ 100 = .00005, a number 10,000 times smaller than .5!

Correct solution:

.5 = 50%   50% means 50/100, which = .5.

There is no question that this answer makes *sense*.

RATIOS

It is stated that the ratio of $5 to $10 is 1:2. A ratio is the same thing as a fraction, so, in this problem, the ratio 1:2 = 1/2. A ratio of 1:2 means one part of two equal parts. Since the one whole debt owed ($10) has two equal parts ($5 and $5), one part of the two equal parts, or 1:2 has been paid—$5 has been paid, so $5 is still owed.

The figuring of ratios is identical with that of fractions. There is little purpose in this differentiation unless one wishes to solve problems by the use of *proportions*.

Proportions

Texts state that a proportion is the expressed equality between two ratios. Therefore, it can be said:

1:2 :: $5:$10

The double colon means "equals." This proportion could also be written as fractions:

1/2 = 5/10

The terms of the proportion are known as the "means," and the "extremes."

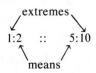

The first and fourth terms are the "extremes," and the second and third terms are the "means." The product of the extremes = the product of the means.

In the proportion 1:2 :: 5:10, the product of the extremes (1×10) equals the product of the means (2×5):

$$1 \times 10 = 2 \times 5$$
$$10 = 10$$

When using proportions to solve problems, usually only three of the four figures are known, and the objective is to figure the unknown quantity that would make an equality. In the problem above, it has been established that the ratio of $5 to $10 is 1:2. To figure what percent this is, proportions can be used:

One ratio, 1:2, is known.

By definition, percent means divided by 100, so 100 is one of the extremes.

x is used for the unknown quantity.

$$1:2 :: x:100$$
$$2x = 100$$
$$x = 100/2 \quad \text{or} \quad 50\%.$$

Therefore $5 is 50% of $10.

Proof:

$$1:2 :: 50:100 \quad \text{OR} \quad 1/2 = 50/100$$

$$\frac{50}{100} = 50\% \qquad\qquad 2 \times 50 = 1 \times 100$$

$$100 = 100$$

The same problem could be solved using fractions, because a ratio is the same thing as a fraction:

$$\frac{1}{2} = \frac{x}{100} \quad \text{OR} \quad \text{Multiply both sides of the}$$

$$2x = 100 \qquad\qquad \text{equation by 100 and reduce the}$$

$$x = 50\% \qquad\qquad \text{fraction (See Appendix).}$$

$$\frac{1}{\cancel{2}} \times \cancel{100}^{50} = \frac{x}{\cancel{100}} \times \cancel{100}$$

$$x = 50\%$$

Summary

Five equivalent ways to express the payment of $5 as part of a $10 debt are:

500¢	1/2	.5	50%	1:2

If these examples do not make sense, the student needs extensive review and drill in the mathematics of fractions and decimal fractions.

USE OF THE TABLE

The table is rearranged because the ratio and fraction are identical. They are placed side by side on the left, and the "cents" column is moved to the extreme right.

1:2	1/2	.5	50%	500¢

The table can now be used to solve problems which follow.

Ten Dollars Owed				
Ratio	Fraction	Decimal	Percent	Cents Paid
1:1	1/1	1.00	100	1,000
1:2	1/2	.5	50	500

Example 1

If 1/100 of the $10 debt has been paid, how many cents have been paid?

Step 1   The fraction 1/100 and its identical ratio are placed in the table. Both of them mean that of the one whole debt owed ($10), one part of 100 equal parts owed has been paid.

Ratio	Fraction	Decimal	Percent	Cents Paid
1:100	1/100			

Step 2   To change 1/100 to a decimal:

$$1/100 \text{ means } 1. \div 100$$

The decimal point is moved two places to the left.

$$1.00 \div 100 = .01 \quad \text{OR} \quad 100 \overline{)1.00}^{.01}$$

This decimal is placed in the table.

Ratio	Fraction	Decimal	Percent	Cents Paid
1:100	1/100	.01		

Step 3   To change .01 to a percent, remember that percent means hundredths, so

.01 is multiplied by 100/100.

The decimal point is moved two places to the right; the denominator 100 is dropped, and a % sign is substituted for it.

$$\begin{array}{r} \% = 100\% \\ \times .01 \\ \hline 1.00\% \end{array} \qquad \text{OR} \qquad \% = .01 \times \frac{100}{100} = 1.\%$$

To simplify the equation, a % sign is substituted for the denominator 100 from the beginning.

$$\% = \frac{1}{\cancel{100}} \times \cancel{100}\% = 1\%$$

Here too the denominator 100 is assumed throughout the equation, and a % sign is substituted for it. This percent is put into the table.

Ratio	Fraction	Decimal	Percent	Cents Paid
1:100	1/100	.01	1	

Step 4   To find the cents paid calculate from any one of the equivalents in the table.

Common Fraction or Ratio: 1/100 of 1,000¢ has been paid.

$$\frac{1}{\cancel{100}} \times 10\cancel{00}¢ = 10¢ \text{ paid}$$

Percent: 1% of 1,000¢ has been paid: 1% means 1/100. Therefore, the equation is the same as for a fraction or ratio.

$$1/\cancel{100} \times 1,0\cancel{00}¢ = 10¢ \text{ paid}$$

Decimal Fraction: .01 of 1,000¢ has been paid.

$$.01 \times 1000¢ = 10¢ \text{ paid}$$

(The decimal point is moved three places to the right.)

The table can now be completed.

Ratio	Fraction	Decimal	Percent	Cents Paid
1:100	1/100	.01	1	10

It will not often be necessary to fill in the entire table to find the answer desired. Just one simple problem will give the answer, as illustrated above.

Example 2

If .2 of the $10 debt has been paid, how many cents have been paid?

Step 1   .2 is put in the decimal column of the table.

Ratio	Fraction	Decimal	Percent	Cents Paid
		.2		

Step 2   To find the fraction, .2 is changed to a fraction. "Two-tenths" is written as the fraction 2/10. Then it is reduced to its lowest terms.

$$2/10 = 1/5 \quad \text{(See Appendix)}.$$

This fraction and its identical ratio are put into the table.

Ratio	Fraction	Decimal	Percent	Cents Paid
1:5	1/5	.2		

The ratio means that of the one whole amount owed, one part of five equal parts owed, or 1:5, has been paid.

Step 3   To find the percent paid remember that percent means hundredths, so:

$$\% = .2 \times \frac{100}{100} = \frac{20}{100} \quad \text{or} \quad 20\%$$

This percent is put into the table.

Ratio	Fraction	Decimal	Percent	Cents Paid
1:5	1/5	.2	20	

Step 4   To find the cents paid figure from any one of the other four equivalents:

Common Fraction or Ratio: 1/5 of 1,000¢ has been paid.

$$\frac{1}{\cancel{5}} \times \cancel{1,000¢}^{\ 200} = 200¢ \text{ paid}$$

Decimal Fraction: .2 of 1,000¢ has been paid.

.2 × 1,000¢ = 200¢ paid

Percent: 20% or 20/100 of 1,000¢ has been paid.

$$\frac{20}{\cancel{100}} \times \cancel{1,000¢} = 200¢ \text{ paid}$$

The table can now be completed. Any one of these simple problems could be used to find the answer.

Ratio	Fraction	Decimal	Percent	Cents Paid
1:5	1/5	.2	20	200

Step 5   Test to see if the table makes sense. 1:5 means that one of five equal parts of the 1000¢ has been paid. Therefore:

$$1,000¢ \div 5 = 200¢ \text{ paid}$$

$$200¢ + 200¢ + 200¢ + 200¢ + 200¢ = 1,000¢$$

When multiplying .2 × 1,000¢, frequently an error is made in placing the decimal point. If it is moved only two places to the right instead of three places, thus:

> .2 × 1,000¢ = 20¢
>
> **WRONG!!!**

the answer then is that only 20¢ has been paid, thus:

$$20¢ + 20¢ + 20¢ + 20¢ + 20¢ = 100¢$$

20¢ is only 1/5 of 100¢, not of 1,000¢. Obviously the answer is wrong because it does not make *sense*!

To prove further that this answer is wrong:

$$\frac{20¢}{1,000¢} = \frac{1}{50}, \quad \text{or one part of 50 equal parts}$$

(should be one part of five parts).

To give an example of another common error, assume that the decimal point in the above problem were moved four places to the right instead of three. The answer would have been:

$$.2 \times 1{,}000\cancel{c} = 2{,}000\cancel{c}$$
$$\text{WRONG!!}$$

How ridiculous to say that a fraction of a number is twice the size of that number! Such an error is obvious. These examples demonstrate the importance of taking great care in placing decimal points. A one-place error to the right makes the answer ten times larger than it should be:

$$.2 = 2. \ \underline{\text{WRONG!!}}$$

A one place error to the left makes the answer ten times smaller than it should be:

$$.2 = .02 \ \underline{\text{WRONG!!}}$$

Imagine what such errors would mean in calculating drug dosages! These types of errors, incidentally, are the most common types made.

Example 3

If 5% of the $10 debt has been paid, how many cents have been paid?

Step 1   The 5% is put into the table.

Ratio	Fraction	Decimal	Percent	Cents Paid
			5	

Step 2   To find the decimal fraction, remember that percent means hundredths, so:

$$5\% = 5/100.$$

$$100\overline{)5.00} \quad \frac{.05}{}$$

An easier way to divide by 100 is to move the decimal point two places to the left:

$$5. \div 100 = .05$$

The decimal is put into the table.

Ratio	Fraction	Decimal	Percent	Cents Paid
		.05	5	

Step 3　To find the cents paid, figure from this decimal:

$.05 \times 1{,}000¢ = 50¢$ (To multiply by 1,000, the decimal point
　　　　　　　　　　　　is moved three places to the right.)

OR　　　　1,000¢
　　　$\times$　.05
　　　50.00¢　paid

Cents paid can also be figured directly from 5%:

5% means 5/100, so $\dfrac{5}{1\not{0}\not{0}} \times 10\not{0}\not{0}¢ = 50¢$ paid

Step 4　Though it is not necessary to fill in more than the cents-paid column to solve the problem, the ratio and fraction are figured for practice:

$$.05 = 5/100 = 1/20 = 1{:}20$$

The table can now be completed.

Ratio	Fraction	Decimal	Percent	Cents Paid
1:20	1/20	.05	5	50

If the fraction had been figured first, the cents paid could also have been reached quickly:

$$5\% = 5/100 = 1/20 \qquad \dfrac{1}{\not{2}\not{0}} \times \overset{50}{1{,}\not{0}\not{0}\not{0}¢} = 50¢$$

Example 4

If $3 of the $10 debt has been paid, what percent has been paid?
Step 1　The $3 (300¢) is put into the table.

Ratio	Fraction	Decimal	Percent	Cents Paid
				300

Step 2　To find the fraction and ratio, remember that 300¢ is a

part of 1,000¢, so it can be expressed as a fraction:

$$\frac{300¢}{1,000¢} = \frac{3}{10}$$

The ratio and fraction columns of the table can be filled in.

Ratio	Fraction	Decimal	Percent	Cents Paid
3:10	3/10			300

Step 3   To find the decimal fraction change the fraction, 3/10, to a decimal fraction by dividing the numerator by the denominator.

$$10\overline{)3.0}^{\,.3} \qquad OR \qquad 3/10 = 3 \div 10 = .3$$

(To divide by 10, the decimal point is moved one place to the left.)

Step 4   To find the percent remember that since percent means hundredths, any one of the other equivalents can be used to find %.

$$\text{Using } 300¢: \quad \frac{300¢}{1,000¢} \times \frac{100}{100} = \frac{30}{100} = 30\%$$

$$\text{Using fraction or ratio:} \quad \frac{3}{10} \times \frac{100}{100} = \frac{30}{100} = 30\%$$

$$\text{Using the decimal fraction:} \quad .3 \times 100/100 = 30/100 = 30\%$$

The table can now be completed.

Ratio	Fraction	Decimal	Percent	Cents Paid
3:10	3/10	.3	30	300

REVIEW

In the problem just completed, 3:10 means that of the $10 owed, three parts of ten equal parts have been paid. Three installments of ten equal installments have been paid. Problems encountered will be expressed in any one of these several equivalent ways, and to solve them the student must be able to go accurately from one expression to another. Much of the time, after a little practice, this can rapidly be done mentally. In a metric money system, or in solving drug problems, it is usually required that one equivalent be changed to another.

Table 1.1 summarizes the previous money problems, plus a few others, so that the relationship between these equivalents can be easily

Table 1.1   Summary of Five Equivalent Ways to
Express Money Transactions

		$10 (1,000¢) Owed		
Ratio	Fraction	Decimal	Percent	Cents Paid
1:1	1/1	1.00	100	1,000
1:2	1/2	.5	50	500
1:5	1/5	.2	20	200
1:10	1/10	.1	10	100
1:100	1/100	.01	1	10
1:20	1/20	.05	5	50
1:1,000	1/1,000	.001	.1	1
3:10	3/10	.3	30	300
1:25	1/25	.04	4	40

read. Any problem based on $10, (or, better expressed for the purposes of this text, 1,000¢), can be solved using this table. If only one component is known, the other four can quickly be calculated.

The following table should now be completed by the student.

	Ratio	Fraction	Decimal	Percent	Cents Paid
		$10 (1,000¢) Owed			
A.	1:40				
B.		2/5			
C.			.0001		
D.				.2	
E.					250

Discussion

A.   The ratio paid is 1:40

Step 1   1:40 means that of the 1,000¢ owed, one of forty equal parts, or 1/40 of the debt, has been paid. Therefore, 1/40 is the fraction.

Step 2   To express 1:40, or 1/40 as a decimal, the numerator is divided by the denominator.

$$\begin{array}{r} .025 \\ 40\overline{)1.000} \\ \underline{80} \\ 200 \\ \underline{200} \end{array}$$

The ratio 1:40 = .025 (a decimal fraction), 25 thousandths.

Step 3   To express 1:40 as a percent, .025 is multiplied by 100/100.

$$.025 \times \frac{100}{100} = \frac{2.5}{100} \quad \text{or} \quad 2.5\%$$

OR

$$\% = .025 \times 100 = 2.5$$

(To multiply by 100, the decimal point is moved two places to the right.)

Step 4   To express 1:40 as cents paid:

$$\frac{1}{\cancel{40}} \times \cancel{1,000}\cancel{\emptyset} = 25\cancel{\emptyset} \quad \text{paid}$$

OR

$$.025 \times 1,000\cancel{\emptyset} = 25\cancel{\emptyset} \quad \text{paid}$$

OR

$$\frac{2.5}{\cancel{100}} \times 1,\cancel{000}\cancel{\emptyset} = 25\cancel{\emptyset} \quad \text{paid}$$

This 25¢ is one part of forty equal parts that make up the whole of 1,000¢. The one part, 25¢, could be expressed as a reduced fraction:

$$\frac{25}{1,000} = \frac{1}{40}$$

B.   The fraction paid is 2/5

Step 1   To express 2/5 as a ratio, remember that any fraction can be converted to a ratio by substituting a colon for the dividing line between the numerator and the denominator. In this problem, the fraction is 2/5, so the ratio is 2:5.

Step 2   To express 2/5 as cents paid, remember that the ratio 2:5 means that of the whole 1,000¢ owed, two of five equal parts have been paid. Therefore, 1,000¢ ÷ 5 = 200¢, the value of each one of the five equal parts. Since two of the five equal parts have been paid, 200¢ is multiplied by 2:

$$200\cancel{\emptyset} \times 2 = 400\cancel{\emptyset} \text{ paid}$$

OR

to solve this problem in one step:

$$\frac{2}{\cancel{5}} \times 1,\cancel{000}\cancel{\emptyset} = 400\cancel{\emptyset} \text{ paid.}$$

Step 3 To express 2/5 as a decimal, divide the numerator by the denominator:

$$2 \div 5 = .4$$

Therefore, of the 1,000¢ owed,

$$.4 \times 1,000¢ = 400¢ \text{ paid.}$$

Step 4 To express 2/5 as a percent remember that since percent means 100/100:

$$\frac{2}{\cancel{5}} \times \frac{\cancel{100}^{20}}{100} = \frac{40}{100} = 40\%$$

Since 40% means $\dfrac{40}{100}$:

$$\frac{40}{\cancel{100}} \times 1,\cancel{000}¢ = 400¢ \text{ paid}$$

C. The decimal paid is .0001

Step 1 To express .0001 as cents paid:

$$.0001 \times 1,000¢ = .1¢ \text{ paid}$$

Step 2 To express .0001 as a percent remember that since percent means hundredths:

$$.0001 \times \frac{100}{100} = \frac{.01}{100} \quad \text{or} \quad .01\%$$

To figure cents paid directly from percent:

$$.01\% \quad \text{or} \quad \frac{.01}{\cancel{100}} \times 1,\cancel{000}¢ = .1¢ \text{ paid}$$

(.1¢ of the 1,000¢ debt has been paid. These figures will be significant in drug problems to be studied in the next chapter.)

Step 3 To express .0001 as a fraction or ratio:

$$.0001 = 1/10,000 \quad \text{or} \quad 1:10,000$$

One of 10,000 equal parts owed has been paid. The decimal is read one ten-thousandth. (See Appendix). ''1'' is the numerator, and ''10,000'' is the denominator.

D. The percent paid is .2%

Step 1 To express .2% as a decimal:

$$.2\% \text{ means } .2/100 \quad \text{or} \quad .2 \div 100, \text{ which} = .002$$

Step 2 To express .2% as cents paid:

.2% or .002 of the 1,000¢ owed, has been paid.

$\frac{.2}{100} \times 1,000¢ = 2¢$ paid or .002 × 1,000¢ = 2¢ paid

Step 3 To express .2% as a fraction or ratio:

.2% = .002 = 2/1,000 = 1/500

The fraction is 1/500, and the ratio is 1:500. 1:500 means that of 500 equal parts, one of them has been paid.

1 ÷ 500 = .002 or .2%

E. 250¢ of the 1,000¢ owed has been paid

Step 1 To express 250¢ as a fraction or ratio:

$\frac{250¢}{1,000¢}$ reduced = 1/4

The fraction 1/4 = a ratio of 1:4

Step 2 To express 250¢ paid as a decimal:

$\frac{250}{1,000} = \frac{1}{4} = 1 ÷ 4 = .25$

Step 3 To express 250¢ as a percent:

$\frac{250}{1,000} \times \frac{100}{100} = \frac{25}{100} = 25\%$

Practice problems with answers follow. Before going to the next chapter, where discussion of drug problems is presented, these practice problems should be studied until the answers are obvious.

PRACTICE PROBLEMS

In all of the problems, assume that $10 (1,000¢) is owed:

1. If $4 of the debt was paid, what percent was paid?
2. If 35% of the debt had been paid, how many cents was paid?
3. If 1/250 of the debt was paid, what percent was paid? How many cents was paid?
4. If 3:5 of the debt was paid, how many cents was this?
5. If 1/20 of the $10 was paid, how can this be expressed as a decimal fraction?
6. If 1:400 of the debt was paid, what percent was this?
7. If $3.50 was paid, how can this be expressed as a ratio?

8. If 20¢ was paid, what is a decimal and a percent that expresses this?
9. If .6% of the debt was paid, how many cents was paid?
10. If 80¢ was paid, what percent of the $10 was this? How can this be expressed as a ratio?

ANSWERS

1. 40% of the debt was paid.
2. 350¢ was paid.
3. 4 cents, or .4% was paid.
4. 600¢ was paid.
5. The decimal is .05.
6. 1:400 = .25%.
7. The ratio is 7:20.
8. The decimal is .02; the percent is 2%.
9. 6¢ has been paid.
10. 80¢ is 8% of $10; the ratio is 2:25.

Chapter 2
MATHEMATICS
OF DRUGS
AND SOLUTIONS

TERMINOLOGY

A few terms commonly used in the math of drugs and solutions must be defined:

1. A *solute* is a substance dissolved in a *solvent* to make a *solution*. A solute may be in the form of a solid, liquid, or gas. It may be "pure" drug, or a concentrated solution.
2. A *solvent* is the component of a solution that is capable of dissolving another substance known as a *solute*.
3. A *solution* is a spontaneously forming homogeneous mixture of two or more substances that do not settle on standing.
4. *Dissolve* means to cause to pass into solution.
5. *Dilute* means to thin or reduce the concentration of a solute, or of a solute in a solution, to lessen the potency, strength, or purity of it by mixing it with more solvent (usually water or saline when used with drugs).
6. A *stock* solution is a relatively concentrated solution from which a weaker solution can be made by diluting it with more solvent (usually water or saline when used with drugs).

Discussion

1. A solute is dissolved in a solvent to make a solution. For example, 5% dextrose in water—dextrose is dissolved in water to make a dextrose solution.
2. A pure drug is 100% drug. In other words, it is an unadulterated substance which exists in solid, liquid, or gaseous form.
3. Solutions can be made from pure drugs, which exist in powder, tablet, liquid, or gaseous form.
4. A 10% solution of a drug used for adults is diluted with water to make a 5% solution for children. The concentration of the solute is thereby thinned or reduced to one-half that of the stock adult solution.

21

METRIC UNITS OF WEIGHT AND VOLUME

If 1 gram (g) of any drug is compared mathematically to 1,000¢, all the relationships will be identical to those figured in Chapter 1. There are 1,000 milligrams (mg) in 1 gram just as there are 1,000¢ in $10.00. The cause of many mathematical errors made in drugs and solutions problems is that people do not remember that "milli" means "thousandths." Therefore, it is imperative to learn that:

1. The kilogram (kg) is the basic unit of weight (or mass) in the metric system. "Kilo" means "thousand," so 1 kilogram = 1,000 grams. The kilogram is so large that it is rarely used for measuring drugs. Often it is used for measuring body weight, or the weight of large specimens, etc.
2. The gram is a unit of weight that is very useful for measuring drug dosages.
3. The milligram is 1/1,000 of a gram and is used extensively for measuring dosages of drugs.
4. The liter (L) is the basic unit for measuring liquids in the metric system.
5. The milliliter (ml) is 1/1,000 of a liter. Milliliters (ml) and cubic centimeters (cc) have the same value, and the two terms can be used interchangeably.

1 kilogram (kg)	= 1,000 grams (g)
1 gram (g)	= 1,000 milligrams (mg)
1 liter (L)	= 1,000 milliliters (ml), or 1,000 cubic centimeters (cc)
1 milligram (mg)	= 1/1,000 gram (g)
1 milliliter (ml), or 1 cubic centimeter (cc)	= 1/1,000 liter (L)

Textbooks state that 1 g (weight) of a solid substance is equal to 1 ml or 1 cc (volume) of that substance. The reason this is so relates to the fact that 1 ml or 1 cc of pure water weighs 1 g at 4°C. Although it is only an approximation to use these terms interchangeably when figuring drugs and solutions problems, it is accurate enough to be safe. Therefore, for this text, assume that

$$1 \text{ g} = 1 \text{ ml} \quad \text{or} \quad 1 \text{ cc}$$

when referring to a pure (100%) drug. If a pure (100%) drug exists in liquid form, then

1 g of that drug is contained in 1 ml.

Pure (100%) drugs may be swallowed as tablets or capsules and occasionally as liquids, generally with a glass of water.

Potent drugs must be greatly diluted with water, saline, or other solvent before being used.

A table similar to the one in Chapter 1 will be used for figuring dilution problems. Only the number of mg/ml desired after dilution, (or the % of the solution) and the total dosage (or total volume of solution) required needs to be known. Notice in the table below that only one column has a different label from those in Chapter 1. The "cents paid" column is now mg/ml (milligrams/milliliter).

Ratio	Fraction	Decimal	Percent	mg/ml	g/L
1:1	1/1	1.00	100	1,000	1,000

Another useful column has been added to this table. Many drugs, particularly intravenous fluids, are given by the liter, and they all have a solute of some sort in them. A very common example is 5% dextrose in water. Therefore, a g/L (grams per liter) column has been added. Since a gram is 1,000 milligrams, and a liter is 1,000 milliliters, both the numerator and the denominator of the mg/ml column have been multiplied by 1,000. Instead of expressing this large amount of drug and solvent as 1,000,000 mg/1,000 ml, it is much more easily read as 1,000 g/L. Therefore, when the term g/L is used, an identical number with that in the "mg/ml" column appears in the g/L column. The table indicates that in any 100% pure liquid drug, there are 1000 mg (or 1 g) in 1 ml, and that there are 1000 g (or 1 kg) of pure drug in 1 L of solvent.

Use of the Table

Problem 1

Make 500 ml of a 50% solution from a 100% pure liquid drug.

Step 1 The table for 100% and 50% solutions is calculated.

Ratio	Fraction	Decimal	Percent	mg/ml	g/L
1:1	1/1	1.00	100	1,000	1,000
1:2	1/2	.5	50	500	500

Step 2 The volume, or number of ml, of the required 50% solution must be known. Generally, this can be determined by the total dosage of drug a doctor orders, or the volume that seems reasonable to accomplish the purpose. For example, a glassful might be required to soak a finger, or a bathtub full to soak the entire body of a burned patient, or 5 ml to be given intravenously, or 1/2 ml to be given

subcutaneously. In this problem it is important to recognize that there must be 500 mg of drug in *each* ml of the solution being prepared. 500 ml of a 50% solution must be made from a 100% liquid drug; 500 mg must be in *each* ml.

Since each ml must contain 500 mg of drug, and 500 ml is the volume required:

$$\begin{array}{r} 500 \text{ mg/ml} \\ \times \quad 500 \text{ ml} \\ \hline 250{,}000 \text{ mg} \end{array}$$

OR

$$\frac{500 \text{ mg}}{\text{ml}} \times 500 \text{ ml} = 250{,}000 \text{ mg} \qquad \text{(See Appendix)}.$$

Step 3   250,000 mg is changed to g.

$$1 \text{ g} = 1000 \text{ mg}$$

Therefore,

$$g = mg \div \frac{1000 \text{ mg}}{g}$$

$$250{,}000 \text{ mg} \div \frac{1000 \text{ mg}}{g} = 250{,}000 \text{ mg} \times \frac{g}{1000 \text{ mg}} \quad \text{(See Appendix)}.$$

$$= 250 \text{ g}$$

250 g of drug is needed to make 500 ml of a 50% solution.

Step 4   Pure (100%) drug is available in liquid form. In a 100% drug, there are 1,000 mg, or 1 g in each ml. A total of 250 g of drug is needed. Since there is 1 g of drug in each ml of the stock drug, 250 ml of stock drug is required. 250 ml of water (or other solvent) is added to make 500 ml total solution.

250 ml stock 100% drug + 250 ml of water = 500 ml total volume.

500 ml of a 50% solution has been made from a stock 100% liquid drug.

This fact could be written:

$$\frac{250 \text{ g}}{500 \text{ ml}}$$

This fraction means that 250 g of drug are contained in 500 ml of solution. Such a fraction is verbally expressed as 250 g per 500 ml.

Step 5   Proof:

$$250 \text{ g} \div 500 \text{ ml} = 250 \text{ g} \times \frac{1}{\underset{2}{500} \text{ ml}} = \frac{1 \text{g}}{2 \text{ml}} \text{ or } \frac{.5 \text{ g}}{\text{ml}}$$

OR

$$\frac{.5 \text{ g/ml}}{500 \text{ ml} \overline{)250.0 \text{ g}}}$$

This only proves that if 250 g of drug is dissolved in a solution whose total volume is 500 ml, each ml contains .5 g, or 500 mg, of drug. The table shows that 500 mg/ml = a 50% solution.

Do these figures make *sense*?

Step 6   Suppose the drug is manufactured in a powder or tablet. 500 ml of a 50% solution must be made:

250 g of the powder or tablets is measured and dissolved in 500 ml of water. Care must be taken that it all dissolves.

Again, 500 ml of a 50% solution would have been made. It would contain 500 mg/ml, or 250 g/500 ml.

Multiplication and Division of g, mg, L, ml

There are several steps in the problem just completed that deserve comment, especially where the terms g, mg, ml, and L, are involved. 500 mg of drug dissolved in 1 ml of water is expressed as the fraction 500 mg/ml. This is a fraction reduced to its lowest terms. (See Appendix).

Notice that

$$\frac{250 \text{ g}}{500 \text{ ml}} = \frac{1 \text{ g}}{2 \text{ ml}} = \frac{.5 \text{ g}}{\text{ml}} \quad \text{or} \quad \frac{500 \text{ mg}}{\text{ml}}$$

The multiplication and division of the units themselves should be discussed because they are used so extensively when figuring drug problems. They are fractions, and therefore, cancellation is usually possible. (See Appendix).

1)
$$\frac{\text{mg}}{\cancel{\text{ml}}} \times \cancel{\text{ml}} = \text{mg}$$

$$\frac{500 \text{ mg}}{\cancel{\text{ml}}} \times 500 \cancel{\text{ml}} = 250,000 \text{ mg}$$

2)
$$\frac{\text{g}}{\cancel{\text{ml}}} \times \cancel{\text{ml}} = \text{g}$$

$$\frac{.5 \text{ g}}{\cancel{\text{ml}}} \times 500 \cancel{\text{ml}} = 250 \text{ g}$$

3)
$$\text{mg} \div \frac{\text{mg}}{\text{ml}} = \cancel{\text{mg}} \times \frac{\text{ml}}{\cancel{\text{mg}}} = \text{ml}$$

$$250,000 \text{ mg} \div \frac{500 \text{ mg}}{\text{ml}} = \overset{500}{\cancel{250,000}} \cancel{\text{mg}} \times \frac{\text{ml}}{\cancel{500 \text{ mg}}} = 500 \text{ ml}$$

This equation indicates that if 250,000 mg of drug is available, and it is desired to dilute it to 500 mg/ml, 500 ml of solvent will be needed.

4)
$$gm \div \frac{g}{ml} = g \times \frac{ml}{g} = ml$$

$$250\ g \div \frac{.5\ g}{ml} = 250\ g \times \frac{500}{.5\ g}\ ml = 500\ ml$$

This equation also shows that, if it is desired to dilute 250 g of drug to .5 g/ml, 500 ml of solvent will be needed. The problems are identical, so the answers are identical. Equivalent terms are used.

5)
$$g \div ml = g \times \frac{1}{ml} = \frac{g}{ml}$$

$$250\ g \div 500\ ml = 250\ g \times \frac{1}{\underset{2}{500}\ ml} = \frac{1\ g}{2\ ml} \quad \text{or} \quad .5\ g/ml$$

This equation shows that, if there are 250 g of drug in 500 ml, there is .5 g in 1 ml.

These problems demonstrate how important it is always to label all parts of an equation, so that the meaning of the answer will be clear. In addition, it must be remembered that in any one equation, figures must all be in the same unit of measure:

If g is used, all weight terms must be in g.
If mg is used, all weight terms must be in mg.
If ml is used, all volume terms must be in ml.
If L is used, all volume terms must be L.

Meaning of the Columns

The table of a 50% solution accompanying problem 1 above shows six equivalent ways to express the amount of drug that is present in a given solution. Any problem that states any one of these six equivalents can quickly be changed or converted to any one of the other equivalents that might be needed to solve the problem. The meaning of each of the columns is discussed below.

The ratio column

Ratio means g/ml. The table of a 50% solution shows that the ratio is 1:2. This means that there is 1 g of drug in each 2 ml of water. Usually it is necessary to know how many mg there are in 1 ml of water (or solvent). If there is 1 g of drug in 2 ml, there are 1,000 mg/2 ml, or 500 mg/ml. The table indicates this equivalent in the mg/ml column. In this manner it is always simple to figure the number of mg/ml directly from the ratio of drug to solvent.

This fact can be illustrated with a practical problem that is a little more complex. Epinephrine is commonly distributed in tiny 1 ml ampoules. The label may indicate only the strength of its contents:

"Epinephrine 1:1000
1 ml"

In an emergency situation, time is a major factor and the dosage of the drug must be figured rapidly and correctly. Perhaps 1/2 mg of epinephrine must be given; all that is known is that there is available 1 ml of a 1:1,000 solution of epinephrine. Since ratio means g/ml, in this instance there is 1 g of epinephrine in 1,000 ml of solvent, or 1,000 mg in 1,000 ml.

$$1,000 \text{ mg}/1000 \text{ ml} = 1 \text{ mg/ml}$$

Since 1/2 mg of epinephrine must be given, 1/2 ml of the drug is administered. It can be said that there is 1 mg/ml of drug in any 1:1,000 solution.

Does this problem make *sense*?

The fraction column

No discussion is needed. The fraction is the same as the ratio, and also means g/ml. The fraction is 1/2, and means 1 g in each 2 ml of solvent, just as the ratio does.

The decimal column

Since a decimal is really a decimal fraction, it also means g/ml. The table shows that a 50% solution = .5. This means that there is .5 g of drug in 1 ml of solution, or .5 g/ml.

$$\frac{.5 \text{ g}}{\text{ml}} \times \frac{1,000 \text{ mg}}{\text{g}} = \frac{500 \text{ mg}}{\text{ml}}$$

Since .5 is also expressed five-tenths or $^5/_{10}$, one might think that there would be 5 g in 10 ml of solvent. This is true. It is the same strength as .5 g/ml.

$$5 \text{ g} \div 10 \text{ ml} = 5 \text{ g} \times \frac{1}{\underset{2}{10 \text{ ml}}} = 1 \text{ g/2 ml, or .5 g/ml}$$

The percent column

Since % means hundredths, this column means g/100 ml. A 50% solution contains 50 g of drug in 100 ml. It should always be remembered that % is a fraction, with the denominator 100 understood. 50% means 50 g/100 ml, so a 50% solution contains 50 g/100 ml of solvent.

Since % means g/100 ml, it can be changed to a decimal by dividing by 100. The decimal point is moved two places to the left in both the numerator and the denominator. The result equals the number of g in 1 ml of solvent.

$$50\% = \frac{50.0 \text{ g} \div 100}{100.0 \text{ ml} \div 100} = \frac{.5 \text{ g}}{1.0 \text{ ml}} \text{ or } .5 \text{ g/ml}$$

The mg/ml column

Mg/ml means just what it says, i.e., the number of mg of drug dissolved in 1 ml of solvent. To get the number of mg/ml present in a 50% solution, it is easiest to change 50% to a decimal, as illustrated above, and multiply the equation by 1,000 mg/g.

$$\frac{.5 \text{ g}}{\text{ml}} \times \frac{1,000 \text{ mg}}{\text{g}} = \frac{500 \text{ mg}}{\text{ml}}$$

OR

$$\frac{50 \text{ g}}{100 \text{ ml}} \times \frac{1,000 \text{ mg}}{\text{g}} = \frac{500 \text{ mg}}{\text{ml}}$$

The g/L column

Earlier it was stated that this column is merely the mg/ml column multiplied by 1,000, and expressed as g/L. The "number" preceding g/L is identical with the "number" preceding mg/ml.

500 mg/ml is an equivalent strength to 500 g/L

Does this statement make *sense*?

Problem 2

Another way to look at problem 1 is to make as much of a 50% solution as is possible from all the existing stock 100% drug.

Step 1 Measure the total amount of stock 100% liquid drug available. Assume there is 75 ml.

Step 2 The % of the stock solution, the % of the solution desired, and the number of ml of stock solution available, are known. They are put into the table thus:

	Percent (g/100 ml)	Decimal (g/ml)
75 ml stock available	100	1.00
Make	50	.5

Step 3   The g/ml of the stock solution is multiplied by the total number of ml of stock solution available. The total amount of drug available will then be known.

$$\frac{1\,g}{ml} \times 75\ ml = 75\ g,\ \text{total amount of drug available.}$$

Step 4   A 50% solution is to be made. Each ml will contain .5 g of drug. The 75 g of drug available is divided by the desired .5 g/ml.

$$75\ g \div \frac{.5\,g}{ml} = \overset{150}{75\ g} \times \frac{ml}{.5\,g} = \begin{array}{l}\text{150 ml, total volume of 50\%}\\ \text{drug that can be made from 75 ml}\\ \text{of 100\% stock drug.}\end{array}$$

Step 5   150 ml is the answer to the problem. All of the 75 ml of stock 100% drug, which contains 1 g/ml, is taken, and water (or other solvent) is added to it to make a total volume of 150 ml. This makes a total of 150 ml of a 50% solution, which contains .5 g/ml.

This solution could also be expressed as

$$75\ g/150\ ml$$

To prove this, 75 g/150 ml is reduced to .5 g/ml, which is a 50% solution.

$$\frac{75\ g}{150\ ml} = 75\ g \div \frac{150\ ml}{1} = \overset{.5}{75}\ g \times \frac{1}{150\ ml} = \frac{.5\ g}{ml} = \frac{500\ mg}{ml}$$

Does this problem make *sense*? If the student is unsure of any of the above calculations, he should review them until they are crystal clear. Effort expended now will really pay off in quick understanding of future chapters.

Problem 3

"Intravenous 5% dextrose in water, 1,000 ml" is very commonly ordered in hospitals. This is a liter of 5% dextrose in water, abbreviated from now on as 5% D/W. The amount of dextrose in this liter of water can be figured by use of the table. Since

$$5\%\ \text{means}\ \frac{5\ g}{100\ ml} = \frac{5000\ mg}{100\ ml}\ ,\ \text{or 50 mg/ml:}$$

Percent	mg/ml	g/L
5%	50	50

Since there are 50 mg in 1 ml of a 5% solution, there are 50 g (or 50,000 mg) of drug in a liter (1,000 ml) of water. The g/L column helps out here.

Problem 4

Fill in the following table. Answers will be found at the end of this chapter. The student is encouraged to make up problems for practice.

Ratio	Fraction	Decimal	Percent	mg/ml	g/L
1:1					
1:10					
1:100					
1:1000					
1:10,000					
1:100,000					
1:2					
1:20					
1:200					
1:2000					
1:20,000					
1:200,000					
2:3					
	4/5				
		.25			
			.4		
				375	
					20
3:8					
	1/50				
		.004			
			20		
				25	
					.1

Problem 5

There are hundreds of drugs manufactured in a 1% concentration. By this time the student should instantly recognize that there are 10 mg/ml in a 1% solution because 1% means 1 g or 1,000 mg/100 ml.

$$1,000 \text{ mg} \div 100 \text{ ml} = 10 \text{ mg/ml}$$

(To divide by 100, move the decimal point two places to the left.)

OR

$$1000 \text{ mg} \div \frac{100 \text{ ml}}{1} = 1,000 \text{ mg} \times \frac{1}{100 \text{ ml}} = 10 \text{ mg/ml}$$

Ratio (g/ml)	Fraction (g/ml)	Decimal (g/ml)	Percent (g/100 ml)	mg/ml	g/L
1:100	1/100	.01	1	10	10

Make 100 ml of a 1% solution.

1% means 1 g/100 ml or 1,000 mg/100 ml = 10 mg/ml

Add 1 g of drug to 100 ml of solvent.

OR

The ratio also gives an instant answer. 1:100 means 1 g/100 ml. If 1 g (1,000 mg) of drug is added to 100 ml of water, 100 ml of a 1% solution has been made. (See table above for equivalents of 1%.)

Problem 6

Make 100 ml of a 1% solution from a 10% solution.
Step 1 A table of 1% and 10% is made.

Ratio (g/ml)	Fraction (g/ml)	Decimal (g/ml)	Percent (g/100 ml)	mg/ml	g/L
1:100	1/100	.01	1	10	10
1:10	1/10	.1	10	100	100

Step 2 100 ml of a 1% solution is wanted. The total amount of drug needed is figured first. A 1% solution contains 10 mg/ml of drug.

$$100 \, ml \times \frac{10 \text{ mg}}{ml} = 1000 \text{ mg, total amount of drug needed.}$$

Step 3 The table shows that a 10% stock solution contains 100 mg/ml. Since 1,000 mg total drug is needed to make 100 ml of a 1% solution, 1,000 mg is divided by 100 mg/ml to determine the volume of stock solution needed.

$$1,000 \text{ mg} \div \frac{100 \text{ mg}}{ml} = 1,\overset{10}{000} \text{ mg} \times \frac{ml}{100 \text{ mg}} = \frac{10 \text{ ml of stock}}{10\% \text{ drug needed.}}$$

Therefore, take 10 ml of a 10% stock solution and add 90 ml of water to make 100 ml of a 1% solution. (Does the answer to this problem make *sense?*)

Problem 7

A 5% solution of a drug is available and 10 ml of a 1% solution must be made from it. Which parts of the table are known, and which parts are needed to solve the problem?

Step 1 The table is made from the information known.

	Percent	mg/ml
Stock drug	5	50
Want 10 ml	1	10

Step 2 The total amount of drug needed is figured first. 10 ml of a solution containing 10 mg/ml is required.

$$\frac{10 \text{ mg}}{\text{ml}} \times 10 \text{ ml} = 100 \text{ mg, total drug needed.}$$

Step 3 The table shows how many mg/ml are contained in the stock 5% solution. 5% = 50 mg/ml. 100 mg total drug is needed.

Stock drug = 50 mg/ml

$$100 \text{ mg} \div \frac{50 \text{ mg}}{\text{ml}} = \overset{2}{100 \text{ mg}} \times \frac{\text{ml}}{50 \text{ mg}}$$

$$= 2 \text{ ml of stock drug needed.}$$

Step 4 2 ml of the 5% stock drug is measured and 8 ml of water is added to make the 10 ml required. 10 ml of a 1% solution with a total dosage of 100 mg/10 ml has been made from a 5% stock solution.

Problem 8

A 10 ml syringe is filled with a 1% solution of a drug. The patient is given 6 ml of it. What total dosage of drug did the patient get?

Step 1

$$1\% = 10 \text{ mg/ml}$$

Step 2 10 mg/ml × 6 ml = 60 mg, total dosage of drug received by the patient.

$$\frac{10 \text{ mg}}{\text{ml}} \times 6 \text{ ml} = 60 \text{ mg}$$

Problem 9

If it is desired to give 20 mg of a drug labeled "1% solution," how many ml should be given?

Step 1 Mg/ml of a 1% solution is figured. The table shows that 1% solutions contain 10 mg/ml.

Step 2   It is desired to give 20 mg.

$$20 \text{ mg} \div \frac{10 \text{ mg}}{\text{ml}} = \overset{2}{\cancel{20 \text{ mg}}} \times \frac{\text{ml}}{\cancel{10 \text{ mg}}} = 2 \text{ ml}$$

2 ml of the drug should be given. (Does this problem make *sense*?)

On the next page, Table 2.1 compares some of the money problems from Chapter 1 with drugs and solutions problems from Chapter 2.

Answers to Problem 4

Ratio	Fraction	Decimal	Percent	mg/ml	g/L
1:1	1/1	1.00	100	1000	1000
1:10	1/10	.1	10	100	100
1:100	1/100	.01	1	10	10
1:1000	1/1000	.001	.1	1	1
1:10,000	1/10,000	.0001	.01	.1	.1
1:100,000	1/100,000	.00001	.001	.01	.01
1:1,000,000	1/1,000,000	.000001	.0001	.001	.001
1:2	1/2	.5	50	500	500
1:20	1/20	.05	5	50	50
1:200	1/200	.005	.5	5	5
1:2000	1/2000	.0005	.05	.5	.5
1:20,000	1/20,000	.00005	.005	.05	.05
1:200,000	1/200,000	.000005	.0005	.005	.005
2:3	2/3	.666	66.6	666	666
4:5	4/5	.8	80.0	800	800
1:4	1/4	.25	25	250	250
1:250	1/250	.004	.4	4	4
3:8	3/8	.375	37.5	375	375
1:50	1/50	.02	2	20	20
3:8	3/8	.375	37.5	375	375
1:50	1/50	.02	2	20	20
1:250	1/250	.004	.4	4	4
1:5	1/5	.2	20	200	200
1:40	1/40	.025	2.5	25	25
1:10,000	1/10,000	.0001	.01	.1	.1

Some of the problems in the latter part of the table repeat some of those in the first part. This has been done intentionally, because it gives the student practice in starting at different columns in the table. For practice, it is suggested that the student figure the mg/ml column for each of the problems directly from the ratio column. Answers should be identical with those originally reached.

Table 2.1 Money Problems Compared with Drugs and Solutions Problems

	Ratio (g/ml)	Fraction (g/ml)	Decimal (g/ml)	Percent (g/100 ml)	Cents Paid or mg/ml
1,000¢ or $10 owed	1:1 = all or whole paid	1/1 = all or whole paid	1.00 = all or whole paid	100% = 100 of 100 equal parts paid	1,000¢ of 1,000¢ paid
1 g or 1,000 mg	1:1 = 1 g/ml	1/1 = 1 g/ml	1.00 = 1 g/ml	100% = 100 g/100 ml	1,000 mg/ml
1,000¢ or $10 owed	1:2 = 1 of 2 equal parts paid	1/2 = 1 of 2 equal parts paid	.5 = .5 of 1,000¢ paid	50% = 50 of 100 equal parts paid	500¢ paid of 1,000¢ owed
1 g or 1,000 mg	1:2 = 1 g/2 ml	1/2 = 1 g/2 ml	.5 = .5 g/ml	50% = 50 g/100 ml	500 mg/ml
1,000¢ or $10 owed	1:4 = 1 of 4 equal parts paid	1/4 = 1 of 4 equal parts paid	.25 = .25 of 1,000¢ paid	25% = 25 of 100 equal parts paid	250¢ paid of 1,000¢ owed
1 g or 1,000 mg	1:4 = 1 g/4 ml	1/4 = 1 g/4 ml	.25 = .25 g/ml	25% = 25 g/100 ml	250 mg/ml

1,000¢ or $10 owed	1:10 = 1 of 10 equal parts paid	1/10 = 1 of 10 equal parts paid	.1 = .1 of 1,000¢ paid	10% = 10 of 100 equal parts paid	100¢ paid of 1,000¢ owed
1 g or 1,000 mg	1:10 = 1 g/10 ml	1/10 = 1 g/10 ml	.1 = .1 g/ml	10% = 10 g/100 ml	100 mg/ml
1,000¢ or $10 owed	1:100 = 1 of 100 equal parts paid	1/100 = 1 of 100 equal parts paid	.01 = .01 of 1,000¢ paid	1% = 1 of 100 equal parts paid	10¢ paid of 1,000¢ owed
1 g or 1,000 mg	1:100 = 1 g/100 ml	1/100 = 1 g/100 ml	.01 = .01 g/ml	1% = 1 g/100 ml	10 mg/ml
1,000¢ or $10 owed	1:20 = 1 of 20 equal parts paid	1/20 = 1 of 20 equal parts paid	.05 = .05 of 1,000¢ paid	5% = 5 of 100 equal parts paid	50¢ paid of 1,000¢ owed
1 g or 1,000 mg	1:20 = 1 g/20 ml	1/20 = 1 g/20 ml	.05 = .05 g/ml	5% = 5 g/100 ml	50 mg/ml
1,000¢ or $10 owed	2:5 = 2 of 5 equal parts paid	2/5 = 2 of 5 equal parts paid	.4 = .4 of 1,000¢ paid	40% = 40 of 100 equal parts paid	400¢ paid of 1,000¢ owed
1 g or 1,000 mg	2:5 = 2 g/5 ml	2/5 = 2 g/5 ml	.4 = .4 g/ml	40% = 40 g/100 ml	400 mg/ml

Chapter 3
PRACTICE

This chapter works with many different kinds of problems that medical personnel encounter. With practice, many of them can be done mentally. *Practice* is the key to the use of this method. Before tackling any medical math problem, the following steps should be followed:

1. State the problem; determine *exactly* what needs to be calculated from available data.
2. Determine which parts of the table are needed for rapid figuring.
3. *Label each* part of *each* calculation to avoid confusion.
4. After each calculation, be sure that the answer makes *sense*.

Discussion follows each problem, but it is suggested that the student try to solve the problems before referring to it. In many of the problems the correct answer can be reached by working with a different part of the table than that used in the discussion, which demonstrates the versatility of the table. The text helps to solve the problems in the most expeditious way.

It is to be hoped that as the student works with these problems, he will begin to see how simple most of them really are. Always be sure that the answers make *sense*.

1. How many mg of a solute are contained in 4 ml of a 20% solution?

$$A\ 20\%\ solution = 20\ g/100\ ml.$$
$$20\ g/100\ ml = .2g/ml$$
$$.2\ g/ml = 200\ mg/ml$$
$$\frac{200\ mg}{ml} \times 4\ ml = 800\ mg$$

It makes *sense*. There are 800 mg/4 ml. A drug containing 200 mg/ml is a 20% solution.

2. A _____% solution is made if 400 mg of a solute are added to 10 ml.

$$\%\ means\ g/100\ ml$$
$$400\ mg/10\ ml = 4,000\ mg/100\ ml\ or\ 4\ g/100\ ml$$
$$4\ g/100\ ml = 4\%$$

3. A _____% solution is made if 12 g of a solute are added to 480 ml.

$$12 \text{ g}/480 \text{ ml} = 1 \text{ g}/40 \text{ ml}$$
$$= .025 \text{ g/ml}$$
$$= 2.5 \text{ g}/100 \text{ ml} = 2.5\%$$

4. A _____% solution is made with 5 mg of a solute in 10 ml.

$$5 \text{ mg}/10 \text{ ml} = 50 \text{ mg}/100 \text{ ml} = .050 \text{ g}/100 \text{ ml}$$
$$.05 \text{ g}/100 \text{ ml} = .05\%$$

5. How many mg of drug are there in 2 ml of a 1:1,000 solution?

ratio means g/ml

$$1:1,000 = 1 \text{ g}/1,000 \text{ ml} = 1,000 \text{ mg}/1,000 \text{ ml} = 1 \text{ mg/ml}$$

Therefore, 2 ml of a 1:1,000 solution contains 2 mg of drug.

6. Many problems contain several different drugs. Each drug's concentration must be figured individually. They cannot be added together. Think of a kettle of water in which 50 apples, 9 oranges, and 1 banana are floating around. It would be ridiculous to say that 50 apples + 9 oranges + 1 banana = 60 lemons. Similarly, if there are 50 g of dextrose, 9 g of sodium chloride, and 1 g of penicillin in a liter of water, the bottle should be labeled:

"5% dextrose in .9% saline + .1% penicillin"

To find the total dosage of each drug;

$$5\% = 5 \text{ g}/100 \text{ ml} = 50 \text{ g of dextrose/L}$$
$$.9\% = .9 \text{ g}/100 \text{ ml} = 9 \text{ g of saline/L}$$
$$.1\% = .1 \text{ g}/100 \text{ ml} = 1 \text{ g of penicillin/L}$$

Here is a typical problem of this nature, used for a spinal anesthetic. After adding 2 ml of a 1% pontocaine solution to 3 ml of 10% dextrose, the concentration of the pontocaine is _____%. The concentration of dextrose is _____%. There are two problems here:

a. Add 2 ml of pontocaine, 1%, to 3 ml of another liquid. The total volume is now 5 ml.

1% pontocaine = 10 mg/ml

$$2 \text{ ml of 1\% pontocaine} = 20 \text{ mg of drug} \left(2 \text{ ml} \times \frac{10 \text{ mg}}{\text{ml}} = 20 \text{ mg} \right)$$

The 20 mg of pontocaine is dissolved in 5 ml of solution.

$$20 \text{ mg}/5 \text{ ml} = 4 \text{ mg}/\text{ml}$$

$$4 \text{ mg}/\text{ml} = 400 \text{ mg}/100 \text{ ml} = .4 \text{ g}/100 \text{ ml}$$

The concentration of the pontocaine is .4%.

b. Add 3 ml of 10% dextrose to 2 ml of another liquid. The total volume is now 5 ml.

$$10\% \text{ dextrose} = 100 \text{ mg}/\text{ml}$$

$$3 \text{ ml of } 10\% \text{ dextrose} = 3 \text{ m\hspace{-0.35em}/l} \times \frac{100 \text{ mg}}{\text{m\hspace{-0.35em}/l}} = 300 \text{ mg}$$

The 300 mg of dextrose is now dissolved in 5 ml of solution.

$$300 \text{ mg}/5 \text{ ml} = 60 \text{ mg}/\text{ml}$$

$$60 \text{ mg}/\text{ml} = 6,000 \text{ mg}/100 \text{ ml} = 6 \text{ g}/100 \text{ ml}$$

The concentration of the dextrose is 6%.

7. A _____% solution is made if 50 g of dextrose is dissolved in 1,000 ml.

$$50 \text{ g}/1,000 \text{ ml} = 5 \text{ g}/100 \text{ ml} = 5\%$$

8. How much drug should be added to 400 ml of water to make a .4% solution?

$$.4\% = .4 \text{ g}/100 \text{ ml}$$

$$\frac{.4 \text{ g}}{100 \text{ ml}} \times 400 \text{ ml} = 1.6 \text{ g}$$

To make a .4% solution, add 1.6 g of drug to 400 ml of water.

9. In 50 ml of a 50% solution there are _____g.

$$50\% = 50 \text{ g}/100 \text{ ml}$$

$$\frac{\overset{25}{50 \text{ g}}}{\underset{2}{100 \text{ ml}}} \times 50 \text{ ml} = 25 \text{ g}.$$

10. In 2 ml of a 2% solution there are _____mg.

$$2\% = 2 \text{ g}/100 \text{ ml} = .02 \text{ g}/\text{ml} = 20 \text{ mg}/\text{ml}$$

$$\frac{20 \text{ mg}}{\text{m\hspace{-0.35em}/l}} \times 2 \text{ m\hspace{-0.35em}/l} = 40 \text{ mg}$$

11. In 180 ml of a 2.5% solution there are _____g.

$$2.5\% = 2.5 \text{ g}/100 \text{ ml} = .025 \text{ g}/\text{ml}$$

$$\frac{.025 \text{ g}}{\text{m\hspace{-0.35em}/l}} \times 180 \text{ m\hspace{-0.35em}/l} = 4.5 \text{ g}$$

12. A _____% solution is made by adding 60 mg of a drug to 2 ml.

$$60 \text{ mg}/2 \text{ ml} = 30 \text{ mg}/\text{ml} = .030 \text{ g}/\text{ml} = 3 \text{ g}/100 \text{ ml} = 3\%$$

13. A _____% solution is made by adding 9 g of a drug to 1,000 ml.

9 g/1,000 ml = .9 g/100 ml = .9% solution

14. How much drug is required to make 1,000 ml of a 2.5% solution?

2.5% = 2.5 g/100 ml = 25 g/1,000 ml

To make a 2.5% solution, add 25 g of drug to 1 L of solvent.

15. How much solvent is added to 1 g of drug to make a 2.5% solution?

2.5% = 2.5 g/100 ml = 25 g/1,000 ml = 1 g/40 ml = 1:40

To make a 2.5% solution, add 40 ml of solvent to 1 g of drug.

16. How much drug is added to 1,000 ml to make a 1% solution?

1% = 1 g/100 ml = 10 g/1,000 ml

To make a 1% solution, add 10 g of drug to 1,000 ml of solvent.

17. How much drug is added to 1,000 ml to make a .1% solution?

.1% = .1 g/100 ml = 1 g/1,000 ml

To make a .1% solution, add 1 g of drug to 1,000 ml of solvent.

18. How much drug is added to 100 ml to make a 1% solution?

1% = 1 g/100 ml

To make a 1% solution, add 1 g of drug to 100 ml of solvent.

19. How much drug is added to 100 ml of solvent to make a .1% solution?

.1% = .1 g/100 ml = 100 mg/100 ml

To make a .1% solution, add 100 mg of drug to 100 ml of solvent.

20. How much drug is added to 600 ml of solvent to make a .2% solution?

.2% = .2 g/100 ml

$$\frac{.2 \text{ g}}{\cancel{100 \text{ ml}}} \times \cancel{600 \text{ ml}}^{6} = 1.2 \text{ g}$$

To make a .2% solution, 1.2 g of drug is added to 600 ml of solvent.

21. How many .1 g tablets are added to 10 ml of solvent to make a 2% solution?

2% = 2 g/100 ml = .2 g/10 ml

Since one tablet contains .1 g of drug

$$.2 \text{ g} \div \frac{.1 \text{ g}}{\text{tablet}} = \cancel{.2 \text{ g}}^{2} \times \frac{\text{tablet}}{\cancel{.1 \text{ g}}} = 2 \text{ tablets}$$

To make a 2% solution, add two tablets (.1 g each) to 10 ml of solvent.

22. A drug is labeled "15 mg/240 ml." If 3 mg of the drug is the desired dosage, how many ml should be given?

$$15 \text{ mg}/240 \text{ ml} = 3 \text{ mg}/48 \text{ ml}$$

In 48 ml of the solution there are 3 mg of the drug. Give 48 ml.

23. If 4 g of drug are added to 400 ml of solvent, how many mg/ml will there be? What % solution will this be?

$$4 \text{ g}/400 \text{ ml} = 4{,}000 \text{ mg}/400 \text{ ml} = 10 \text{ mg/ml}$$

$$4 \text{ g}/400 \text{ ml} = 1 \text{ g}/100 \text{ ml} = 1\% \text{ solution}$$

24. Prepare 4 L of a 1:20 solution.

1:20 means 1 g/20 ml

$$\frac{1 \text{ g}}{\cancel{20} \text{ ml}} \times \overset{200}{\cancel{4{,}000} \text{ ml}} = 200 \text{ g}$$

To make a 1:20 solution, add 200 g of drug to 4 L of solvent.

25. Make 1 L of a 1% solution. 1% means 1 g/100 ml, or 10 g/1,000 ml. To make a 1% solution, add 10 g of drug to 1,000 ml of solvent.

26. Make 1 L of a 1:25 solution.

1:25 means 1 g/25 ml

$$\frac{1 \text{ g}}{\cancel{25} \text{ ml}} \times \overset{40}{\cancel{1{,}000} \text{ ml}} = 40 \text{ g}$$

To make a 1:25 solution, add 40 g of drug to 1 L of solvent.

27. Make 500 ml of a .5% solution.

.5% means .5 g/100 ml

$$\frac{.5 \text{ g}}{\cancel{100} \text{ ml}} \times \overset{5}{\cancel{500} \text{ ml}} = 2.5 \text{ g}$$

To make a .5% solution, add 2.5 g of drug to 500 ml of solvent.

28. Make 200 ml of a 4% solution. 4% means 4 g/100 ml, or 8 g/200 ml. To make a 4% solution, add 8 g of drug to 200 ml of solvent.

29. How many .2-g tablets are needed to make 500 ml of a 1:2,000 solution?

$$1{:}2{,}000 = 1 \text{ g}/2{,}000 \text{ ml} = .5 \text{ g}/1{,}000 \text{ ml} = .25 \text{ g}/500 \text{ ml}$$

$$.25 \text{ g} \div \frac{.2 \text{ g}}{\text{tablet}} = \overset{1.25}{\cancel{.25} \text{ g}} \times \frac{\text{tablet}}{\cancel{.2} \text{ g}} = 1.25 \text{ tablets}$$

To make a 1:2,000 solution, add 1.25 tablets (.2 g each) to 500 ml of solvent.

30. How much drug is required to make 1 L of a 1:1,000 solution? 1:1,000 means 1 g/1,000 ml. To make 1 L of a 1:1,000 solution, add 1 g of drug to 1 L of solvent.

31. How much drug is needed to make 100 ml of a 10% solution? 10% means 10 g/100 ml. To make 100 ml of a 10% solution, add 10 g of drug to 100 ml of solvent.

32. Make 500 ml of a 1:5,000 solution. 1:5,000 means 1 g/5,000 ml, or .1 g/500 ml. To make 500 ml of a 1:5,000 solution, add .1 g (100 mg) of drug to 500 ml of solvent.

33. Make 2 L of a 3% solution. 3% means 3 g/100 ml, or 30 g/1,000 ml, or 60 g/2,000 ml. To make 2 L of a 3% solution, add 60 g of drug to 2 L of solvent.

34. How much of a 10% solution is needed to make 500 ml of a 5% solution? 10% means 10 g/100 ml, or .1 g/ml. 5% means 5 g/100 ml.

$$\frac{5\ g}{100\ ml} \times \overset{5}{500\ ml} = 25\ g\ \text{total drug needed}$$

$$25\ g \div .1\ g/ml = \overset{250}{25\ g} \times \frac{ml}{.1\ g} = 250\ ml$$

To make 500 ml of a 5% solution, add 250 ml of a 10% solution to 250 ml of solvent.

35. How much of a 1:5 solution is needed to prepare 500 ml of a 10% solution?

$$10\% = 10\ g/100\ ml$$

$$\frac{10\ g}{100\ ml} \times \overset{5}{500\ ml} = 50\ g\ \text{total drug needed}$$

1:5 means 1 g/5 ml

$$50\ g \div 1\ g/5\ ml = 50\ g \times \frac{5\ ml}{1\ g} = 250\ ml\ \text{total 1:5 drug needed}$$

To make 500 ml of a 10% drug, add 250 ml of solvent to 250 ml of stock 1:5 drug.

36. How much of a 5% solution is needed to make 500 ml of a 10% solution? This is an impossible situation. Unless water is distilled off to concentrate the drug, it cannot be done because stronger solutions cannot be made from weaker solutions.

37. How much solvent is needed to make 4 L of a 3% solution from a 10% solution?

10% means 10 g/100 ml, or 100 g/L

3% means 3 g/100 ml, or 30 g/L

$$\frac{30 \text{ g}}{\cancel{L}} \times 4 \cancel{L} = \begin{array}{l} 120 \text{ g total drug needed to make} \\ 4 \text{ L of a 3% solution} \end{array}$$

$$120 \text{ g} \div \frac{100 \text{ g}}{L} = \overset{1.2}{\cancel{120}} \cancel{\text{g}} \times \frac{L}{\cancel{100} \cancel{\text{g}}} = 1.2 \text{ L}$$

To make 4 L of a 3% solution, add 1.2 L of 10% stock drug to 2.8 L of solvent (1.2 L + 2.8 L = 4 L).

38. How many ml of a 20% solution would be needed to prepare 60 ml of a 4% solution?

20% means 20 g/100 ml = .2 g/ml

4% means 4 g/100 ml or .04 g/ml

$$\frac{.04 \text{ g}}{\cancel{ml}} \times 60 \cancel{ml} = \begin{array}{l} 2.4 \text{ g total drug needed to make} \\ 60 \text{ ml of a 4% solution} \end{array}$$

$$2.4 \text{ g} \div \frac{.2 \text{ g}}{ml} = \overset{12}{\cancel{2.4}} \cancel{\text{g}} \times \frac{ml}{\cancel{.2} \cancel{\text{g}}}$$

$$= 12 \text{ ml of 20% drug needed}$$

Measure 12 ml of 20% stock drug and add 48 ml of solvent. There will be 2.4 g of drug in 60 ml, or .04 g/ml, which is a 4% solution (4 g/100 ml).

39. How much of a 1:5 stock drug is needed to make 4 L of a 1:20 solution?

$$1:20 = 1 \text{ g}/20 \text{ ml}$$

$$\frac{1 \text{ g}}{\cancel{20 \text{ ml}}} \times \overset{200}{\cancel{4,000 \text{ ml}}} = 200 \text{ g total drug needed}$$

$$1:5 = 1 \text{ g}/5 \text{ ml}$$

$$200 \text{ g} \div 1 \text{ g}/5 \text{ ml} = 200 \cancel{\text{g}} \times \frac{5 \text{ ml}}{1 \cancel{\text{g}}}$$

$$= 1000 \text{ ml or 1 L stock 1:5 drug needed}$$

To make 4 L of a 1:20 solution, measure 1 L of the 1:5 stock drug, and add 3 L of solvent.

40. How much of a 25% stock drug is needed to prepare 300 ml of a 1:25 solution?

$$25\% = 25 \text{ g}/100 \text{ ml}$$

$$1:25 = 1 \text{ g}/25 \text{ ml}$$

$$\frac{1 \text{ g}}{25 \text{ ml}} \times \overset{12}{300 \text{ ml}} = \begin{array}{l} 12 \text{ g total drug needed to make} \\ 300 \text{ ml of a } 1:25 \text{ solution} \end{array}$$

$$12 \text{ g} \div 25 \text{ g}/100 \text{ ml} = 12 \text{ g} \times \frac{\overset{4}{100} \text{ ml}}{25 \text{ g}} = 48 \text{ ml}$$

To make 300 ml of a 1:25 solution, measure 48 ml of the stock 25% drug, and add 252 ml of solvent to it.

41. How much of a 12% drug could be made from 30 ml of a 20% drug?

$$20\% = 20 \text{ g}/100 \text{ ml}$$

$$\frac{\overset{1}{20} \text{ g}}{\underset{5}{100} \text{ ml}} \times \overset{6}{30} \text{ ml} = 6 \text{ g total drug available}$$

$$12\% = 12 \text{ g}/100 \text{ ml}$$

$$6 \text{ g} \div 12 \text{ g}/100 \text{ ml} = 6 \text{ g} \times \frac{\overset{50}{100} \text{ ml}}{\underset{2}{12} \text{ g}} = 50 \text{ ml}$$

Measure the 30 ml of stock 20% drug, and add 20 ml of solvent. There will be 6 g/50 ml, or 12 g/100 ml (12%).

42. How much stock solution 1:3 is needed to make 150 ml of a 1:5 solution?

$$1:3 = 1 \text{ g}/3 \text{ ml}$$

$$1:5 = 1 \text{ g}/5 \text{ ml, or } .2 \text{ g/ml}$$

$$\frac{.2 \text{ g}}{\text{ml}} \times 150 \text{ ml} = 30.0 \text{ g total drug needed}$$

$$30 \text{ g} \div 1 \text{ g}/3 \text{ ml} = 30 \text{ g} \times \frac{3 \text{ ml}}{1 \text{ g}} = 90 \text{ ml}$$

To make 150 ml of a 1:5 solution, measure 90 ml of a 1:3 stock drug, and add 60 ml of solvent to it. A 1:5 solution that has .2 g of drug in each ml will have been made.

43. How much of a 3% solution is used to prepare 1,500 ml of a 1:10,000 solution?

$$3\% = 3 \text{ g/100 ml}$$

$$1:10,000 = 1 \text{ g/10,000 ml} = .0001 \text{ g/ml}$$

$$\frac{.0001 \text{ g}}{\cancel{ml}} \times 1,500 \; \cancel{ml} = .15\cancel{00} \text{ g drug needed}$$

$$.15 \text{ g} \div 3 \text{ g/100 ml} = \overset{.05}{\cancel{.15}} \, \cancel{g} \times \frac{100 \text{ ml}}{\cancel{3} \, \cancel{g}}$$

$$= 5 \text{ ml stock drug needed}$$

To make 1,500 ml of a 1:10,000 solution, add 5 ml of stock 3% drug to 1,495 ml of solvent.

44. Prepare .008 g from a 1:50 solution.

$$1:50 = 1 \text{ g/50 ml}$$

$$.008 \text{ g} \div 1 \text{ g/50 ml} = .008 \; \cancel{g} \times \frac{50 \text{ ml}}{1 \; \cancel{g}}$$

$$= .4 \text{ ml stock drug needed}$$

To give .008 g of drug, measure .4 ml of a 1:50 stock solution.

45. Make a 1:20 solution from 200 ml of a 20% solution.

$$20\% = \begin{array}{l} 20 \text{ g/100 ml, or } 40 \text{ g/200 ml,} \\ \text{total stock drug available} \end{array}$$

$$1:20 = 1 \text{ g/20 ml}$$

$$40 \text{ g} \div 1 \text{ g/20 ml} = 40 \; \cancel{g} \times \frac{20 \text{ ml}}{1 \; \cancel{g}} = 800 \text{ ml}$$

To make a 1:20 solution, add 600 ml of solvent to 200 ml of stock 20% solution. There will be 40 g/800 ml.

46. Make 10 ml of a 2% topical spray from 10% stock drug.

$$2\% = 20 \text{ mg/ml}$$

$$\frac{20 \text{ mg}}{\cancel{ml}} \times 10 \; \cancel{ml} = 200 \text{ mg total drug needed}$$

$$10\% = 100 \text{ mg/ml concentration of stock drug}$$

$$200 \text{ mg} \div 100 \text{ mg/ml} = \overset{2}{\cancel{200}} \; \cancel{mg} \times \frac{ml}{\cancel{100 \; mg}} = 2 \text{ ml}$$

To make 10 ml of a 2% spray, measure 2 ml of 10% stock drug, and add 8 ml of solvent to it.

47. Make 30 ml of a 1% drug from 2.5% stock solution.

$$2.5\% = 25 \text{ mg/ml}$$

$$1\% = 10 \text{ mg/ml}$$

$$\frac{10 \text{ mg}}{\text{ml}} \times 30 \text{ ml} = 300 \text{ mg total drug needed}$$

$$300 \text{ mg} \div 25 \text{ mg/ml} = \cancel{300}^{\,12} \text{ mg} \times \frac{\text{ml}}{\cancel{25} \text{ mg}}$$

$$= 12 \text{ ml stock drug needed}$$

To make 30 ml of a 1% drug, measure 12 ml of stock 2.5% solution, and add 18 ml of solvent.

48. Make 1,000 ml of a 1:1,000 solution.

$$1:1,000 = 1 \text{ g}/1,000 \text{ ml}$$

Add 1 g of drug to a liter of solvent.

49. Make 30 ml of a 4% solution from a 20% stock drug.

$$4\% = 4 \text{ g}/100 \text{ ml}$$

$$\frac{4 \text{ g}}{100 \text{ ml}} \times 30 \text{ ml} = 120 \text{ g}/100 = 1.2 \text{ g total drug needed}$$

$$20\% = 20 \text{ g}/100 \text{ ml}$$

$$1.2 \text{ g} \div 20 \text{ g}/100 \text{ ml} = 1.2 \text{ g} \times \frac{\cancel{100}^{\,5} \text{ ml}}{\cancel{20} \text{ g}}$$

$$= 6 \text{ ml total stock drug needed}$$

To make 30 ml of a 4% solution, measure 6 ml of stock 20% drug, and add 24 ml of solvent.

50. The patient was receiving an intravenous infusion of 5% D/W. It was discontinued after he had absorbed only 650 ml of the 1,000 ml bottle. How much dextrose did he get?

$$5\% = 5 \text{ g}/100 \text{ ml}$$

$$\frac{5 \text{ g}}{\cancel{100} \text{ ml}} \times \cancel{650}^{\,6.5} \text{ ml} = 32.5 \text{ g total drug absorbed}$$

Chapter 4
MORE PRACTICE: REAL PROBLEMS THAT MAY BE ENCOUNTERED

Occasionally the dosage of a drug is given according to a patient's weight, which is still usually recorded in pounds. Until all hospitals weigh patients in kilograms, pounds will have to be converted to kilograms. This is not difficult to do if one knows that

$$2.2 \text{ pounds (lb)} = 1 \text{ kilogram (kg)}$$

1. The child's weight is 33 pounds. He is to receive a drug that is commonly given at a dose of 80 mg/kg of body weight. The drug is labeled "1 g = 1 ml," and is to be given in a 2.5% solution. List the steps in preparing this medication.

   a. The metric weight of the child is computed.

   $$33 \text{ lb} \div 2.2 \text{ lb/kg} = \overset{15}{\cancel{33 \text{ lb}}} \times \frac{\text{kg}}{\cancel{2.2 \text{ lb}}} = 15 \text{ kg}$$

   b. The child weighs 15 kg. He is to receive 80 mg/kg of his body weight.

   $$\frac{80 \text{ mg}}{\cancel{\text{kg}}} \times 15 \cancel{\text{kg}} = 1200 \text{ mg, or } 1.2 \text{ g, total dosage}$$

   c. The drug is labeled "1 g = 1 ml."

   $$1.2 \text{ g} \div 1 \text{ g/ml} = 1.2 \cancel{\text{g}} \times \frac{\text{ml}}{1 \cancel{\text{g}}}$$
   $$= 1.2 \text{ ml stock (100\%) drug required}$$

   c. The drug is to be given in a 2.5% solution.

   $$2.5\% = 2.5 \text{ g}/100 \text{ ml}$$
   $$1.2 \text{ g} \div 2.5 \text{ g}/100 \text{ ml} = 1.2 \cancel{\text{g}} \times \frac{\overset{40}{\cancel{100 \text{ ml}}}}{\cancel{2.5 \text{ g}}} = 48.0 \text{ ml}$$

d. Measure 1.2 ml of the stock drug and add enough solvent to make 48 ml.
e. Proof

$$1.2 \text{ g}/48 \text{ ml} = .025 \text{ g/ml} = 2.5 \text{ g}/100 \text{ ml} = 2.5\% \text{ solution}$$

The child receives 80 mg/kg of his body weight (15 kg) in the 48 ml of this 2.5% solution.

2. Sometimes a drug is given according to the patient's weight in pounds. The child's weight is 39 lb. He is to receive a drug that is commonly given at a dose of 15 mg/lb of body weight in a 10% solution. Available are 5-g ampoules of powdered drug. How much total drug should be given to this child?

$$39 \text{ lb} \times \frac{15 \text{ mg}}{\text{lb}} = 585 \text{ mg total drug dosage}$$

List the steps in preparing this medication:
a. 10% = 10 g/100 ml = 5 g/50 ml. Add 50 ml of solvent to the 5-g ampoule of powder. A 10% solution will be made.
b. Since 585 mg is the dosage of the drug to be given and since there are 100 mg/ml in the prepared 10% solution:

$$585 \text{ mg} \div 100 \text{ mg/ml} = \overset{5.85}{\cancel{585} \text{ mg}} \times \frac{\text{ml}}{\cancel{100 \text{ mg}}} = 5.85 \text{ ml}$$

c. The child should receive 5.85 ml of this 10% solution. He will have received 585 mg of the drug, which is 15 mg/lb of his body weight (39 lb).

3. How much sodium chloride is there in 1,500 ml of .85% saline solution?

$$.85\% = .85 \text{ g}/100 \text{ ml} = 8.5 \text{ g/L}$$

$$1,500 \text{ ml} = 1.5 \text{ L}$$

$$\frac{8.5 \text{ g}}{\cancel{L}} \times 1.5 \cancel{L} = \begin{array}{l} 12.75 \text{ g sodium chloride in 1,500 ml} \\ \text{of .85\% saline solution} \end{array}$$

4. The patient's blood pressure is falling rapidly. An intravenous infusion of neosynephrine, .002%, is indicated. The neosynephrine ampoule is a 1% solution. How should this medication be prepared? Available in stock are 1,000-ml, 500-ml, and 250-ml bottles of 5% D/W for use in mixing this drug. How much of this 1% neosynephrine should be added to each bottle to make a .002% solution?

a.   1,000 ml bottle of 5% D/W

$.002\% = .002$ g/100 ml $= 2$ mg/100 ml

$$\frac{2 \text{ mg}}{100 \text{ ml}} \times 1{,}000 \text{ ml} = 20 \text{ mg neosynephrine required}$$

$$1\% = 10 \text{ mg/ml}$$

$$20 \text{ mg} \div 10 \text{ mg/ml} = \overset{2}{\cancel{20 \text{ mg}}} \times \frac{\text{ml}}{\cancel{10 \text{ mg}}}$$

$$= 2 \text{ ml stock neosynephrine required}$$

To make a .002% solution of neosynephrine, add 2 ml of 1% stock neosynephrine to 1,000 ml 5% D/W. (This is the practical answer to this problem. To be absolutely accurate, 2 ml should be removed from the 1,000-ml 5% D/W bottle and the 20 mg of neosynephrine should be added to the remaining 998 ml of 5% D/W. This degree of accuracy is not necessary, and is rarely practiced.)

b.   500-ml bottle of 5% D/W

$$\frac{2 \text{ mg}}{100 \text{ ml}} \times 500 \text{ ml} = 10 \text{ mg neosynephrine required}$$

There are 10 mg/ml in a 1% solution, so 1 ml of this 1% stock neosynephrine solution is added to the 500 ml bottle of 5% D/W. A .002% solution of neosynephrine will have been made.

c.   250-ml bottle of 5% D/W

$$\frac{2 \text{ mg}}{100 \text{ ml}} \times \overset{2.5}{\cancel{250 \text{ ml}}} = 5 \text{ mg neosynephrine required}$$

$$5 \text{ mg} \div 10 \text{ mg/ml} = \overset{.5}{\cancel{5 \text{ mg}}} \times \frac{\text{ml}}{\cancel{10 \text{ mg}}} = .5 \text{ ml}$$

Add .5 ml of 1% stock neosynephrine to 250 ml of 5% D/W to make a .002% solution of neosynephrine.

These three answers all make sense in relation to each other. The 250-ml bottle should be adequate to get the patient through most crises.

5.   Because a patient suffered a cardiac arrest a doctor added one 4-ml ampoule of .2% levophed, to the remaining 400 ml of the patient's bottle of intravenous 5% D/W that was already running.

a.   How many mg/ml of levophed will there be in the resulting solution? What percent solution is this?

$$.2\% = .2 \text{ g}/100 \text{ ml} = .002 \text{ g/ml} = 2 \text{ mg/ml}$$

$$\frac{2 \text{ mg}}{\text{ml}} \times 4 \text{ ml} = 8 \text{ mg total drug per ampoule of levophed}$$

Therefore 8 mg of levophed was added to 400 ml of 5% D/W.

8 mg/400 ml = .02 mg/ml of levophed in the resulting solution

.02 mg/ml = 2 mg/100 ml = .002 g/100 ml = .002% levophed solution

b. If 300 ml of this solution were absorbed by the patient, and then discontinued, how much levophed would the patient have gotten?

$$300 \text{ ml} \times \frac{.02 \text{ mg}}{\text{ml}} = 6.00 \text{ mg}$$

The patient received 6 mg of levophed. (This makes *sense* because the patient received 6 of 8 available mg of the levophed, or three-fourths of the ampoule. He also received 300 ml of the remaining 400 ml of 5% D/W in the intravenous bottle, or three-fourths of that solution.)

c. How should the bottle be labeled after the levophed is added?

"levophed .02 mg/ml; 8 mg/400 ml"

Labeling it in this way, there will be no confusion concerning total dosage of levophed absorbed when the medication is discontinued.

6. Prepare 1,000 ml of 5% alcohol in 5% D/W for intravenous use. Available are 1,000-ml bottles of 5% D/W, and vials of absolute alcohol, which is considered to be a 100% drug (for purposes of calculation).

$$5\% = 5 \text{ g}/100 \text{ ml} = 50 \text{ g/L total dosage of alcohol required}$$

100% drug = 100 g/100 ml = 1 g/ml

$$50 \text{ g} \div 1 \text{ g/ml} = 50 \text{ g} \times \frac{\text{ml}}{\text{g}}$$

$$= 50 \text{ ml absolute alcohol required}$$

Add 50 ml of absolute alcohol to 950 ml of 5% D/W. (This volume of drug is so large that it is practical to remove 50 ml of the 5% D/W before adding the alcohol. Most 1,000-ml bottles of intravenous fluids do not have room enough for an additional 50 ml of drug. Of course, the concentration of the dextrose in water is diluted by adding the alcohol to it.)

7. Make a .2% succinylcholine solution in 5% D/W. Succinylcholine powder in 1-g ampoules, and 5% D/W in 500-ml bottles are available.

.2% means .2 g/100 ml

$$\frac{.2 \text{ g}}{100 \text{ ml}} \times \overset{5}{500 \text{ ml}} = 1.0 \text{ g}$$

To make a .2% succinylcholine solution, add 1 g (one ampoule) of the powdered drug to 500 ml of 5% D/W.

8. Make a .2% succinylcholine solution from vials labeled "20 mg/ml; 10 ml vial." The available solvent is 5% D/W in 500-ml bottles.

$$\frac{20 \text{ mg}}{ml} \times \frac{10 \text{ ml}}{\text{vial}} = 200 \text{ mg/vial total amount of drug in one vial}$$

$$.2\% = .2 \text{ g}/100 \text{ ml} = .002 \text{ g/ml} = 2 \text{ mg/ml}$$

$$2 \text{ mg/ml} \times 500 \text{ ml} = 1{,}000 \text{ mg, or } 1 \text{ g drug required.}$$

$$1{,}000 \text{ mg} \div 200 \text{ mg/vial} = \overset{5}{1{,}000 \text{ mg}} \times \frac{\text{vial}}{200 \text{ mg}}$$

$$= 5 \text{ vials of drug needed to make } 1 \text{ g}$$

To make a .2% solution, add five vials of succinylcholine labeled "20 mg/ml, 10 ml vial," to 450 ml of 5% D/W.

9. Special "cartridges" of xylocaine and epinephrine are available for dentists to use for local anesthesia. To fit the dentist's special type of syringe, all the cartridges contain a volume of 1.8 ml. One such cartridge is labeled:

"Xylocaine 2%

Epinephrine 1:50,000

1.8 ml size"

a. How much xylocaine does this cartridge contain?

$$2\% = 20 \text{ mg/ml}$$

$$\frac{20 \text{ mg}}{ml} \times 1.8 \text{ ml} = 36 \text{ mg total amount of}$$
xylocaine in the cartridge

b. How much epinephrine does this cartridge contain?

$$1:50{,}000 = 1{,}000 \text{ mg}/50{,}000 \text{ ml} = 1 \text{ mg}/50 \text{ ml} = .02 \text{ mg/ml}$$
$$\frac{.02 \text{ mg}}{ml} \times 1.8 \text{ ml} = .036 \text{ mg total amount of}$$
epinephrine contained in the cartridge

10. Another dental cartridge is labeled:

"Carbocaine 2%

Levonordefrin 1:20,000

1.8 ml size"

   a. How much carbocaine does it contain?

2% = 20 mg/ml

20 mg/ml × 1.8 ml = 36 mg of carbocaine in the cartridge

   b. How much levonordefrin does it contain?

1:20,000 = 1,000 mg/20,000 ml = 1 mg/20 ml = .05 mg/ml

.05 mg/ml × 1.8 ml = .090 mg total levonordefrin in the cartridge

11. The label on the ampoule reads ".25 g pentobarbital, 5-ml ampoule." The desired dosage is 25 mg of pentobarbital to be given intravenously. How much of this ampoule should be given to the patient?

.25 g = 250 mg

The ampoule contains 250 mg/5 ml, or 50 mg/ml.

$$25 \text{ mg desired} \div 50 \text{ mg/ml} = 25 \text{ mg} \times \frac{\text{ml}}{\underset{2}{50 \text{ mg}}} = 1/2 \text{ ml}$$

Give .5 ml of the drug. Since there are 50 mg/ml, there are 25 mg/.5 ml.

12. Give prostigmine 1 mg. Available are:
   a. Prostigmine 1:4,000, 2-ml ampoules
   b. Prostigmine 1:2,000, 2-ml ampoules
   c. Prostigmine 1:1,000, 5-ml ampoules
   Using each one of the available ampoules, figure how much of each ampoule should be given to the patient, in order to give 1 mg of prostigmine.
   a. 1:4,000, 2-ml ampoules:

1:4,000 = 1,000 mg/4,000 ml = 1 mg/4 ml

   In a 1:4,000 strength prostigmine solution, 4 ml contains 1 mg of drug. Each ampoule has a volume of 2 ml. Give two ampoules of "prostigmine 1:4,000, 2-ml ampoule."
   b. 1:2,000, 2-ml ampoules:

1:2,000 = 1,000 mg/2,000 ml = 1 mg/2 ml

   In a 1:2,000 strength prostigmine solution, 2 ml contains 1

mg of drug. Each ampoule has a volume of 2 ml. Give one ampoule of "prostigmine 1:2,000, 2-ml ampoule."

c. 1:1,000, 5-ml ampoules:

$$1:1,000 = 1,\cancel{000}\ mg/1,\cancel{000}\ ml = 1\ mg/ml$$

In a 1:1,000 strength prostigmine solution, 1 ml contains 1 mg of drug. Each ampoule has a volume of 5 ml. Give 1 ml from the 5-ml ampoule of prostigmine 1:1,000.

13. Make 20 ml of epinephrine 1:200,000. Available are 1-ml ampoules of 1:1,000 epinephrine, and 50-ml vials of saline.

$$1:200,000 = 1,\cancel{000}\ mg/200,\cancel{000}\ ml = 1\ mg/200\ ml = .005\ mg/ml$$

$$\frac{.005\ mg}{\cancel{ml}} \times 20\ \cancel{ml} = .1\ mg\ total\ epinephrine\ needed$$

Stock epinephrine $1:1,000 = 1,\cancel{000}\ mg/1,\cancel{000}\ ml = 1\ mg/ml = .1\ mg/.1\ ml$. Add .1 ml of epinephrine 1:1,000 to 20 ml of saline. A 1:200,000 solution of epinephrine will have been made.

14. What percent is a 1:200,000 solution?

$$1:200,000 = .005\ mg/ml = .5\ mg/100\ ml = .0005\ g/100\ ml = .0005\%$$

15. A patient received 25 ml of a drug labeled "2% xylocaine with epinephrine 1:100,000."
a. How much xylocaine did he receive?

$$2\% = 20\ mg/ml$$

$$20\ mg/\cancel{ml} \times 25\ \cancel{ml} = 500\ mg\ total\ dosage\ of\ xylocaine\ received$$

b. How much epinephrine did he receive?

$$1:100,000 = 1,\cancel{000}\ mg/100,\cancel{000}\ ml = 1\ mg/100\ ml = .01\ mg/ml$$

$$.01\ mg/\cancel{ml} \times 25\ \cancel{ml} = .25\ mg\ total\ dosage\ of\ epinephrine\ received$$

16. Added to the remaining 125 ml of a 5% D/W infusion is 1 g calcium gluconate.
a. How many mg/ml of calcium gluconate is made?

$$1,000\ mg/125\ ml = 8\ mg/ml$$

b. What percent of calcium gluconate has been made?

$$8\ mg/ml = .008\ g/ml = .8\ g/100\ ml = .8\%$$

c. How much dextrose is there in the 125 ml?

$$5\% = 50\ mg/ml$$

$$50\ mg/\cancel{ml} \times 125\ \cancel{ml} = 6250\ mg = 6.25\ g$$

17. The patient is to receive an intravenous infusion of 1,000 ml of 10% D/W.
    Available is:

    5% D/W, 1,000 ml

    50% D/W, 50-ml ampoules

How can an approximate 10% solution be made?

    10% D/W = 10 g/100 ml

    = 100 g/L total drug needed in 1,000 ml of 10% D/W

    5% D/W = 5 g/100 ml

    = 50 g/L total drug already in the 5% D/W 1,000-ml bottle

    50% D/W = 50 g/100 ml = 25 g/50-ml ampoule

    Add two ampoules of 50% D/W (100 ml) to 900 ml of 5% D/W.

This answer is not exact, but is close enough for most purposes for which this concentration of dextrose is used.

18. Nembutal, 10 mg, is to be given intravenously to a child.
    Available is nembutal .25 g/5-ml ampoule. How should this medication be prepared?

    .25 g/5 ml = 250 mg/5 ml = 50 mg/ml

As it is manufactured, this drug is too concentrated for intravenous use, especially in a child. It should be diluted so that it is easy to give 10 mg of nembutal accurately. There are several ways this can be done. A satisfactory way would be to add to 1 ml (50 mg) of the ampoule enough saline to make 10 ml. Then there would be 50 mg/10 ml or 5 mg/ml.

$$10 \text{ mg} \div 5 \text{ mg/ml} = \overset{2}{\cancel{10} \text{ mg}} \times \frac{\text{ml}}{\cancel{5} \text{ mg}} = 2 \text{ ml}$$

To receive 10 mg of nembutal, this child should receive 2 ml of the nembutal solution which has been diluted to 5 mg/ml.

19. If 1 ml of 1% pontocaine is added to 1 ml of 10% dextrose in preparation for a spinal anesthetic, what is the percent and mg/ml that will result for each drug?
    a. The pontocaine problem:
       1% = 10 mg/ml
       After adding 1 ml of 1% pontocaine to 1 ml of another solution, there will be 10 mg of pontocaine/2 ml or 5 mg/ml.
       5 mg/ml = .5% pontocaine solution

b. The dextrose problem:
    $10\% = 100$ mg/ml
    After adding 1 ml of 10% dextrose to 1 ml of another solution, there will be 100 mg of dextrose/2 ml, or 50 mg/ml.
    50 mg/ml = 5% dextrose solution

20. It is generally accepted that the maximum amount of xylocaine that any patient should receive in one dosage is 7.5 mg/kg of body weight. Under halothane anesthesia, epinephrine should be limited to .1 mg in any 20-minute period and should not be more concentrated than a 1:100,000 solution (Katz's rule for avoiding drug interaction). Available is a 20-ml vial labeled "Xylocaine 2% with epinephrine 1:100,000." How much of this drug would be safe to give in a 20-minute period to a 154-lb patient who is under halothane anesthesia? Which drug is the limiting factor?

$$1 \text{ kg} = 2.2 \text{ lb}$$

$$154 \text{ lb} \div 2.2 \text{ lb/kg} = \overset{70}{\cancel{154\text{ lb}}} \times \frac{\text{kg}}{\cancel{2.2\text{ lb}}}$$

$$= 70 \text{ kg metric weight of the patient}$$

$$70 \cancel{\text{ kg}} \times \frac{7.5 \text{ mg}}{\cancel{\text{kg}}} = 525 \text{ mg maximum safe dose of xylocaine}$$

$$2\% \text{ xylocaine} = 20 \text{ mg/ml}$$

$$525 \text{ mg} \div 20 \text{ mg/ml} = \overset{26.2}{\cancel{525 \text{ mg}}} \times \frac{\text{ml}}{\cancel{20 \text{ mg}}}$$

$$= 26.2 \text{ ml maximum volume of 2\% xylocaine}$$
a 70-kg patient should receive
in any one dosage

$$1:100,000 \text{ epinephrine} = 1,000 \text{ mg}/100,000 \text{ ml or } .01 \text{ mg/ml}$$

$$.1 \text{ mg total allowed} \div .01 \text{ mg/ml} = \overset{10}{\cancel{.1 \text{ mg}}} \times \frac{\text{ml}}{\cancel{.01 \text{ mg}}}$$

$$= 10 \text{ ml of drug allowed}$$
in 20 minutes

The epinephrine limits the amount of this combined drug that should be given in a 20-minute period; 10 ml of it may be given. Wait 20 minutes before giving another 10 ml. After another 20 minutes, another 6 ml may be given, but then the maximum amount of xylocaine (26 ml) will have been given, and no more of the drug would be safe to give during that particular anesthetic.

SECTION TWO

MATHEMATICAL COMPUTATIONS INVOLVED IN BIOCHEMISTRY

Chapter 5
TERMINOLOGY

The mathematics commonly used in biochemistry frightens some students, but there is no reason for this. As with the exercises and problems in Section One, the mathematics of body chemistry involves understanding *exactly* what each term means, and practicing with each one.

TERMS USED IN BIOCHEMISTRY

Common terms useful in body chemistry that will be discussed in this text are:

Physiology
Biochemistry
Atom, Compound, Molecule
Electrolyte
Ion, Cation, Anion
Radical
Acids, Bases, Salts
Homeostasis
Acid-base Balance

Physiology

Physiology is the study of how the body "works." It is the biological science of all the functions, activities, and processes that take place in a living organism.

Biochemistry

The prefix "bio" means life or living organism, so biochemistry is the chemistry of the functions or activities of living organisms. Sometimes biochemistry is called physiological chemistry, because many physiological processes involve biochemical changes of some type.

Atom, Compound, Molecule

An atom is the smallest unit of an element, and it cannot be broken down further (except by atomic fission). Atoms, in nature, are simple, indivisible, and indestructible units that are the basic components of the entire universe.

A compound is a substance consisting of atoms or ions of two or more different elements in definite proportions; it usually has properties unlike those of its constituent elements.

A molecule is the simplest structural unit that displays the characteristic physical and chemical properties of a particular compound.

Electrolytes

Understanding the nature of electrolytes is fundamental to understanding the biochemistry of the living body. The term electrolyte sounds like the word electricity. The living body is an electrical organism that has been described as a leather bag filled with an electrolyte solution. To understand what an electrolyte is, it must first be recognized that there are two ways the molecules of chemical compounds act in solution.

1. The molecules in solution may ionize, i.e., split or dissociate to form ions. This process is known as ionization, and chemical compounds that behave in this way are known as electrolytes. An example of an electrolyte in body water is sodium chloride, ordinary table salt. In chemical symbols, salt is written as NaCl. NaCl ionizes to form sodium ions Na^+ and chloride ions Cl^-. In chemical symbols, this reaction is written as follows:

$$NaCl \rightarrow Na^+ + Cl^-$$

2. If the molecules in the solution remain intact, i.e., undissociated, they do not ionize in the body under any circumstances. Such compounds are known as non-electrolytes. Examples of non-electrolytes which are in solution in the body are dextrose and urea.

Ions, Cations, Anions

Each ion carries either a positive (+) or a negative (−) electrical charge. For example, when sodium chloride (NaCl) is dissolved in water, it dissociates (or ionizes or splits) into sodium ions which have a positive charge (Na^+) and into chloride ions which have a negative charge (Cl^-). The molecule NaCl dissociates into $Na^+ + Cl^-$.

The positive ions are known as cations (pronounced "cat-eye-on"), and the negative ions are known as anions (pronounced "an-eye-on").

If an NaCl solution is made in a flask, the NaCl ionizes and the Na^+ and Cl^- ions dissolve into the solution. If both electrodes of a battery are put into the NaCl solution, and a light bulb is included in the electrical circuit, the light bulb will illuminate.

Figure 5.1 is a schematic representation of the relation between an electrolyte solution such as sodium chloride and a light bulb. If an

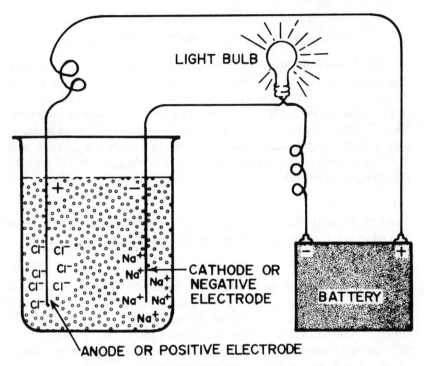

Figure 5.1. Electrical Current Carried by a NaCl Solution

electric current is applied, the current is conducted through the solution, the electrical circuit is completed, and the light bulb glows. During this process, the positive sodium ions (cations) migrate to the negative electrode (cathode), and the negative chloride ions (anions) migrate to the positive electrode (anode).

Therefore, an electrolyte solution is a solution in which the molecules of its solute split into ions, and can carry an electrical current. If, however, the solution in the flask in Figure 5.1 were a non-electrolyte, such as dextrose in water, the current would not be conducted by the solution, and the light bulb would not illuminate.

Types of electrolytes

Strong electrolytes are generally inorganic compounds that are excellent conductors of electricity. They ionize almost completely in an aqueous (water) solution. In other words, they readily dissociate into ions, and so are available to carry a current. Examples of strong electrolytes are:

Hydrochloric acid (HCl) $HCl \rightarrow H^+ + Cl^-$

| Sulfuric acid (H_2SO_4) | $H_2SO_4 \rightarrow 2\,H^+ + (SO_4)^{--}$ |
| Sodium chloride (NaCl) | $NaCl \rightarrow Na^+ + Cl^-$ |

Weak electrolytes are usually organic compounds that are poor conductors of electricity. They only partially dissociate, or do not dissociate at all depending upon the pH of the solution. (The concept of pH is discussed in Chap. 11.) But for now it is enough to remember the difference between strong and weak electrolytes. An example of a very important organic, weak electrolyte in the body is carbonic acid H_2CO_3. It weakly dissociates into only 1 hydrogen ion H^+ and the bicarbonate radical $(HCO_3)^-$.

$$H_2CO_3 \rightarrow H^+ + (HCO_3)^-$$

Most of the carbonic acid stays in the molecular form H_2CO_3 when placed in water. Only a small part of it ionizes.

Radical

Sometimes groups of atoms cling together and act in chemical reactions as if they were really only one ion. Such groups of atoms are known as radicals. An example of the radical $(HCO_3)^-$ was just mentioned. Other common radicals are $(OH)^-$ and $(SO_4)^{--}$. Notice how radicals are enclosed in parentheses and how the sign of the charge (+ or −) and the number of charges are indicated.

Acids, Bases, and Salts

An *acid* is a compound made up of hydrogen and some other element or radical. Two examples of acids are:

| Hydrochloric acid | $H^+ + Cl^- \rightarrow HCL$ |
| Carbonic acid | $H + (HCO_3)^- \rightarrow H_2CO_3$ |

A *base* is a compound made up of a metal, or the ammonium radical, combined with the hydroxyl radical $(OH)^-$. It can generally be said that a compound that will neutralize an acid is a base (sometimes called an alkali). Some examples of bases are:

Sodium hydroxide	$Na^+ + (OH)^- \rightarrow NaOH$
Ammonium hydroxide	$(NH_4)^+ + (OH)^- \rightarrow NH_4OH$
Hydrochloric acid plus sodium hydroxide makes salt (NaCl) and water.	$HCl + NaOH \rightarrow NaCl + HOH$

(The base NaOH neutralizes the acid HCl, and a salt is formed.)

A *salt* is a compound formed by replacing the hydrogen of an acid by a metal or the ammonium radical.

$$HCl + NaOH \rightarrow NaCl + HOH$$
$$HCl + NH_4OH \rightarrow NH_4Cl + HOH$$

Water is commonly expressed as either H_2O or HOH.

Homeostasis

Literally, homeostasis means a static, constant state. When an organism is in a state of equilibrium, maintained by a balance of all chemical and physiological functions, it is said to be in a homeostatic state. In life, the body works constantly to maintain a physiological equilibrium of all its functions, including the concentration of specific electrolytes. When it is successful in maintaining this equilibrium the organism is healthy; when it fails to maintain this equilibrium, the organism is sick.

Nature requires that all organisms live in an electrical world. An electrical current is a series of infinite numbers of electrons that carry a negative charge. They are negative charges with one objective: to find positive charges as "mates." When a negative ion comes into contact with a positive ion, neutralization occurs. The attraction of negative ions for positive ions is extremely strong, as is evidenced by an electrical storm. The negative charges in a thunder cloud are instantly neutralized after a flash of lightning, because they find an infinite source of positive charges in the ground. The heat caused by the speed of the negative electrons causes the air to burn. This burning air is seen as a flash of lightning.

Every movement and function of a living body involves an electrical current of ions seeking "mates" for neutralization. Thus, electrical balance or neutrality is maintained in the body. The *total number of positive charges always equals the total number of negative charges*. Since all organisms live in an electrical world, this neutralization process of all ions takes place constantly in every plant, animal, insect, or other form of life, as well as in the laboratory, and between inanimate objects.

An extremely important function of homeostasis within the body is to maintain *specific* concentrations of each cation and each anion. The healthy body maintains itself within specific, sometimes extremely narrow, ranges of concentrations of each cation and each anion, at all times. When one (or more) of these electrolytes exceeds its normal concentration or becomes deficient in it, the body is sick.

Acid-base Balance

Electrolytes are acids, bases, or salts that dissociate into ions. A great many of them play vital roles in body chemistry. They must be main-

Table 5.1 Plasma Electrolytes Expressed as Milliequivalents/liter (mEq/L)

Cations	mEq/L	Anions	mEq/L
Sodium Na$^+$	142	Bicarbonate (HCO$_3$)$^-$	24
Potassium K$^+$	5	Chloride Cl$^-$	105
Calcium Ca^{++}	5	Phosphate (HPO$_4$)$^{--}$	2
Magnesium Mg^{++}	2	Sulfate (SO$_4$)$^{--}$	1
		(Organic acid)$^-$	6
		Protein Pr$^-$	16
	154 mEq/L		154 mEq/L

154 mEq/L cations = 154 mEq/L anions

tained by the body in specific concentrations. For example, Table 5.1 shows the specific concentrations of electrolytes that are normal for blood plasma.

Many of the different cations and anions can combine with each other to form various compounds of acids, bases, or salts, but the total milliequivalents per liter of each one of them existing in the plasma must remain within a narrow range of the values shown on Table 5.1. The concentrations of other fluid compartments in the body must also be maintained within a very narrow range.

Biochemists refer to this body function as *acid-base balance*. To understand exactly how the body maintains acid-base balance, it is essential to learn to work with equivalent weights, and milliequivalent weights, the subject of the next two chapters.

Chapter 6
EQUIVALENT
WEIGHTS

In Section One it was seen that g/L and mg/ml are the commonly used units for the measurement of drugs and solutions. Unfortunately these units are inadequate for expressing the body's concentrations of electrolytes.

The number of mg/ml of an electrolyte solution yields no information regarding its potential for maintaining electrical neutrality within the body. A method is needed to count the number of ions or number of molecules that exist in a solution. Their individual gram weight is of no consequence. The number of cations that are available to neutralize the same number of anions must be known.

A frequently used analogy illustrates the importance of understanding the difference between gram weights and equivalent weights. Suppose a party were given for a few couples. Would 1,000 pounds of men and 1,000 pounds of women be invited? Ridiculous! How would the hostess know that she had invited an equivalent number of men and women? It would be much better to invite 10 men and 10 women, ignoring what each one weighed. Then the hostess would be sure that she had invited an equivalent number of men and women. To extend this analogy further, think of positive ions (cations) as men, and negative ions (anions) as women. Some men (cations) desire only one mate (anion) at a time, and vice versa. They are "monogamous" or conventional. The chart below lists them as "good" solid citizens.

"Good Men" (cations)	"Good Women" (anions)
H^+ (hydrogen)	Cl^- (chloride)
Na^+ (sodium)	$(OH)^-$ (hydroxyl radical)
K^+ (potassium)	$(HCO_3)^-$ (bicarbonate radical)

The chart shows that H^+ can mate with Cl^- to make HCl (hydrochloric acid) or H^+ can mate with $(OH)^-$ to make HOH or H_2O (water) or H^+ can mate with $(HCO_3)^-$ to make H_2CO_3 (carbonic acid). It shows similarly that:

$$Na^+ + Cl^- \rightarrow NaCl \text{ (sodium chloride)}$$

$$Na^+ + (OH)^- \rightarrow NaOH \text{ (sodium hydroxide)}$$

$$Na^+ + (HCO_3)^- \rightarrow NaHCO_3 \text{ (sodium bicarbonate)}$$

and that:

$$K^+ + Cl^- \rightarrow KCl \text{ (potassium chloride)}$$

$$K^+ + (OH)^- \rightarrow KOH \text{ (potassium hydroxide)}$$

$$K^+ + (HCO_3)^- \rightarrow KHCO_3 \text{ (potassium bicarbonate)}.$$

It would be very easy for chemists if all cations and anions made "good monogamous marriages," desiring only one "mate" at a time. However, such is not the case. Many cations and anions are "bigamists" or "polygamists," requiring two or more "mates" at the same time.

"Polygamists"

Ca^{++} (calcium)	O^{--} (oxygen)	$(SO_4)^{--}$ (sulfate)
Mg^{++} (magnesium)	$(HPO_4)^{--}$ (acid phosphate)	$(CO_3)^{--}$ (carbonate)
Fe^{+++} (iron)	$(PO_4)^{---}$ (phosphate)	S^{--} (sulfur)

VALENCE

From the analogy just discussed, the concept of valence can be understood. A difference in the number of ions that will combine to form molecules of different compounds is illustrated by the following chemical compounds:

$$HCl \quad H_2O \quad CH_4 \quad Fe_2O_3$$

One ion of chlorine combines with one ion of hydrogen to form HCl, but one ion of oxygen combines with two ions of hydrogen to make H_2O. One ion of carbon combines with 4 hydrogen ions.

If an element will combine with hydrogen, the number of hydrogen ions combining with one ion of that element is said to be the valence of that element. In the above examples, the valence of chlorine is 1, oxygen 2, and carbon 4.

Example 1

But Fe_2O_3 is different. There are no hydrogen ions in this compound. Therefore, the number of positive charges that exist in its molecule must be equated with the number of hydrogen ions that would be necessary to replace them. The table of "polygamists" shows that Fe^{+++} is a cation that requires three "mates" at the same time.

Fe^{+++} has a valence of 3, i.e., it is one cation with 3 positive charges. Comparing this ion with H^+, which has a valence of 1, it can be seen that one ion of Fe^{+++} is "worth" three hydrogen ions in its ability to neutralize negative charges.

In this example, Fe^{+++} wants to combine with O^{--} which has a valence of 2.

$$Fe^{+++} + O^{--} \rightarrow ?$$

Looking at the valences involved, it is obvious that if two ions of Fe^{+++} are combined with three ions of O^{--}, all five ions will be satisfied:

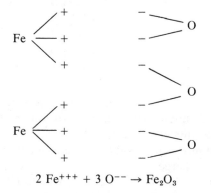

$$2\ Fe^{+++} + 3\ O^{--} \rightarrow Fe_2O_3$$

The subscript indicates the number of ions of an element in a chemical compound, as illustrated. The valence of a cation multiplied by its subscript must be equal to (be *equivalent* to) the valence of its anion multiplied by its subscript:

$$2\ Fe^{+++} \times 3\ \text{positive charges} = 6$$

$$3\ O^{--} \times 2\ \text{negative charges} = 6$$

The number of positive charges equals the number of negative charges. The equation is balanced.

Example 2

Valence is the number of positive or negative charges held by an ion of an element, and it is indicated by the number of $+$ or $-$ signs after the chemical symbol for that element.

$$Ca^{++} + (SO_4)^{--} \rightarrow CaSO_4$$

This is a satisfactory "marriage" because both ions are satisfied. One cation with a valence of 2 has "mated" with one anion that also has a valence of 2. A complete neutralization has occurred, and one molecule of the compound $CaSO_4$ has been formed. Another similar example is:

$$Ca^{++} + (CO_3)^{--} \rightarrow CaCO_3$$

However, if Ca^{++} wants to "mate" with the "good, monogamous girl," chloride, Ca^{++} becomes a "bigamist," and is satisfied only if it "mates" with two chloride atoms at the same time.

$$Ca^{++} + 2\,Cl^- \rightarrow CaCl_2$$

$$Ca \Big\langle \begin{array}{l} + \quad - \!-\!Cl \\ \\ + \quad - \!-\!Cl \end{array}$$

Notice how the equation is written. When there is more than one ion needed to form a compound, the number of ions needed is indicated by the subscript, in this case $CaCl_2$.

Again, the number of positive charges must *always* equal the number of negative charges.

To sum up, Ca^{++} has a valence of 2, which means that each ion of calcium possesses 2 positive charges; Cl^- has a valence of 1, which means that each ion of chloride possesses 1 negative charge. Therefore, to form the compound calcium chloride, two ions of chloride are needed to neutralize one ion of calcium, thereby forming one molecule of calcium chloride.

Example 3

Na^+, K^+, and H^+ can combine with the radicals $(SO_4)^{--}$ or $(CO_3)^{--}$. Both radicals require two "mates."

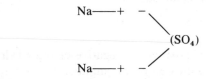

$$Na \!-\!\!-\! + \quad - \searrow \atop {(SO_4)} \atop Na \!-\!\!-\! + \quad - \nearrow$$

Two Na^+ ions are needed to satisfy "bigamist" $(SO_4)^{--}$. One molecule of Na_2SO_4 is made.

$$K \!-\!\!-\! + \quad - \searrow \atop {(SO_4)} \atop K \!-\!\!-\! + \quad - \nearrow$$

One molecule of K_2SO_4 is made.
Similarly:

$$2\,Na^+ + (CO_3)^{--} \rightarrow Na_2CO_3$$

$$2\,K^+ + (CO_3)^{--} \rightarrow K_2CO_3$$

$$2\,H^+ + (CO_3)^{--} \rightarrow H_2CO_3$$

The $(CO_3)^{--}$ radical also requires 2 "mates."

Example 4

Na———+   –
                           (CO_3)

H———+   –

$$Na^+ + H^+ + (CO_3)^{--} \rightarrow NaHCO_3$$

Here 1 Na^+ ion and 1 H^+ ion unite with the $(CO_3)^-$ radical to neutralize it, and one molecule of sodium bicarbonate is formed. The equation is balanced, because 2 positive charges have combined with 2 negative charges.

Similarly, in each instance below, three positive ions neutralize three negative ions, or radicals:

$$2\,Na^+ + H^+ + (PO_4)^{---} \rightarrow Na_2HPO_4 \text{ (sodium phosphate)}$$

$$Na^+ + 2\,H^+ + (PO_4)^{---} \rightarrow NaH_2PO_4 \text{ (sodium acid phosphate)}$$

$$2\,K^+ + H^+ + (PO_4)^{---} \rightarrow K_2HPO_4 \text{ (potassium phosphate)}$$

$$K^+ + 2\,H^+ + (PO_4)^{---} \rightarrow KH_2PO_4 \text{ (potassium acid phosphate)}$$

Examples of the way calcium combines:

$$Ca^{++} + 2\,Cl^- \rightarrow CaCl_2 \text{ (calcium chloride)}$$

$$Ca^{++} + 2\,(OH)^- \rightarrow Ca(OH)_2 \text{ (calcium hydroxide)}$$

$$Ca^{++} + 2(HCO_3)^- \rightarrow Ca(HCO_3)_2 \text{ (calcium bicarbonate)}$$

GRAM EQUIVALENT WEIGHTS

Equivalent means equal valence. An equivalent weight (commonly called an equivalent) measures or counts the *number of charges*, not the gram weight. This fact is the key to understanding the entire concept of "counting" in equivalent weights.

The ability of one cation of an element (or of a radical) to replace one hydrogen cation in a molecule, or the ability of one anion of an element (or of a radical) to combine with one hydrogen cation to make a molecule is known as the chemical combining ability, or the chemical combining power, of that element. Hydrogen ionizes to H^+; it has only one positive charge. Table 6.1 shows that one gram atomic weight of hydrogen weighs only 1 g, the least amount of any of the elements. For these two reasons, hydrogen was chosen as the element with which all other elements are compared.

Although one ion of each of the elements weighs more in grams than does one ion of hydrogen, the relative weights are *not* concerned with the combining ability of the element. It is the *number of charges* (positive or negative) possessed by one ion of an element that *is* concerned when comparing *its* combining ability with that of one ion of hydrogen.

An equivalent weight of an element is its weight in grams that is equivalent or equal in combining ability to that of 1 g of hydrogen. It is the total gram weight of the number of ions of an element that is equal in combining ability to the number of ions that are in 1 g of hydrogen. (See *Avogadro's Number, p. 73*.)

Table 6.1   Common Gram Atomic Weights and Valences

Element	Symbol	Gram Atomic Weight	Valence
Bromine	Br	80	$-1, -3, -5, -7$
Calcium	Ca	40	$+2$
Carbon	C	12	$+4, -4$
Chlorine	Cl	35	-1
Hydrogen	H	1	$+1$
Iron	Fe	56	$+2, +3$
Magnesium	Mg	24	$+2$
Nitrogen	N	14	$+3, +5$
Oxygen	O	16	-2
Potassium	K	39	$+1$
Phosphorus	P	31	$+3, +5$
Sodium	Na	23	$+1$
Sulfur	S	32	$-2, +4, +6$

Radicals			
Ammonium	NH_4		$+1$
Bicarbonate	HCO_3		-1
Carbonate	CO_3		-2
Chlorate	ClO_3		-1
Hydroxyl	OH		-1
Nitrate	NO_3		-1
Phosphate	PO_4		-3
Sulfate	SO_4		-2

The atomic weight of an element, expressed in grams, as illustrated in Table 6.1, is called the *gram atomic weight* (GAW) of that element. Using hydrogen, which has a GAW of 1, as a standard, all other elements have GAWs relative to, or compared with, that of hydrogen.

The molecular weight of a compound, expressed in grams, is called the *gram molecular weight* (GMW) of the compound, and it is the sum of the GAWs of all atoms present in the molecule. One GMW is commonly known as 1 mol or 1 mole.

Definition of Gram Equivalent Weight

The *gram equivalent weight* (GEW) of an element (or radical) is the *number* of gram atomic weights, or the *fraction* of one gram atomic weight of that element, that exactly combines with, or exactly replaces 1 GAW of hydrogen.

Illustration 1

$$1 \text{ GAW } Cl^- + 1 \text{ GAW } H^+ \rightarrow 1 \text{ GMW HCl}$$

(To make 1 GMW HCl, combine 1 GAW of Cl^-

with 1 GAW of H^+.)

By definition, it can be seen that, since 1 GAW of Cl^- combines exactly with 1 GAW of H^+, the GEW of Cl^- is the same as its GAW.

$$1 \text{ GAW (35 g) } Cl^- + 1 \text{ GAW (1 g) } H^+ \rightarrow 1 \text{ GMW (36 g) HCl}$$
$$1 \text{ GEW (35 g) } Cl^- + 1 \text{ GEW (1 g) } H^+ \rightarrow 1 \text{ GEW (36 g) HCl}$$

Therefore:

$$1 \text{ GEW } Cl^- = 1 \text{ GAW } Cl^-$$

(Both of them weigh 35 g and so are identical.)

$$1 \text{ GEW } H^+ = 1 \text{ GAW } H^+$$

(Both of them weigh 1 g and so are identical.)

Illustration 2

$$1 \text{ GAW } Na^+ + 1 \text{ GMW HCl} \rightarrow 1 \text{ GMW NaCl} + 1 \text{ GAW } H^+$$

(To form the salt, 1 GAW of the element Na^+,

which has a valence of +1, replaces 1 GAW of H^+.)

By definition, since 1 GAW of Na^+ exactly replaces 1 GAW of H^+, the GEW of Na^+ is the same as its GAW.

$$1 \text{ GAW } (23 \text{ g}) \text{ Na}^+ + 1 \text{ GMW } (36 \text{ g}) \text{ HCl}$$

$$\rightarrow 1 \text{ GMW } (58 \text{ g}) \text{ NaCl} + 1 \text{ GAW } (1 \text{ g}) \text{ H}^+$$

$$1 \text{ GEW } (23 \text{ g}) \text{ Na}^+ + 1 \text{ GEW } (36 \text{ g}) \text{ HCl}$$

$$\rightarrow 1 \text{ GEW } (58 \text{ g}) \text{ NaCl} + 1 \text{ GEW } (1 \text{ g}) \text{ H}^+$$

Therefore:

$$1 \text{ GEW Na}^+ = 1 \text{ GAW Na}^+$$

(Both of them weigh 23 g, and so are identical.)

Illustration 3

$$1 \text{ GAW S}^{--} + 2 \text{ GAW H}^+ \rightarrow 1 \text{ GMW H}_2\text{S}$$

Sulfur presents a different situation. Table 6.1 indicates that S^{--} has a valence of 2, requiring two "mates" at the same time. Hydrogen requires only one "mate." Since sulfur is a "bigamist," one ion of H^+ can satisfy only half of one sulfur ion. Therefore, the GEW of S^{--} (the amount that can combine exactly with 1 GAW of H^+) equals the GAW of sulfur divided by 2. The general rule for calculating the GEW of any element is:

$$\text{GEW} = \frac{\text{GAW}}{\text{valence}}$$

Table 6.1 shows that the GAW of S^{--} is 32 g, and that it has a valence of 2.

$$\text{GEW of } S^{--} = \frac{32 \text{ g}}{2} = 16 \text{ g}$$

By definition, it can be seen that the GEW of sulfur is the fraction of its GAW that combines exactly with 1 GAW of H^+. The GEW of S^{--} equals its GAW/2, because only half of a sulfur ion will combine with one ion of hydrogen.

$$1 \text{ GAW } (32 \text{ g}) \text{ S}^{--} + 2 \text{ GAW } (2 \text{ g}) \text{ H}^+ \rightarrow 1 \text{ GMW } (34 \text{ g}) \text{ H}_2\text{S}$$

$$1 \text{ GEW } (16 \text{ g}) \text{ S}^{--} + 1 \text{ GEW } (1 \text{ g}) \text{ H}^+ \rightarrow 1 \text{ GEW } (17 \text{ g}) \text{ H}_2\text{S}$$

Note: *1 GEW* of S^{--} + *1 GEW* H^+ → *1 GEW* H_2S

AVOGADRO'S LAW AND NUMBER

Avogadro's Law

Equivalent weights can be completely understood if the significance of Avogadro's law is recognized. Avogadro's law states that one GMW (which is the sum of the GAW of all the atoms present in a molecule) of any compound contains the same *number* of molecules as one GMW of any other compound. Similarly, one GAW of any element contains the same *number* of atoms as one GAW of any other element.

Example

In 1 GAW of Na^+ (which weighs 23 g) there are the same *number* of ions as 1 GAW of Cl^- (which weighs 35 g)

OR

In 1 GAW of H^+ (which weighs 1 g) there are the same *number* of ions as 1 GAW of Na^+ (which weighs 23 g), or of Cl^- (which weighs 35 g), etc.

Also:

The *number* of molecules in 1 GMW of H_2SO_4 is the same as in 1 GMW of H_2CO_3.

The weight of 1 GMW of H_2SO_4 is 98 g. To get this weight, the GAW of each of its components are added $(1 + 1 + 32 + 16 + 16 + 16 = 98$ g$)$.

The weight of 1 GMW of H_2CO_3 is 62 g $(1 + 1 + 12 + 16 + 16 + 16 = 62$ g$)$.

To go back to the analogy of the party, ''men'' and ''women'' are being counted, not how much each one weighs. So, 1 GAW of chlorine (35 g of ''girl'') ''marries'' 1 GAW of hydrogen (1 g of ''boy''), to make 1 GMW of HCl.

Avogadro's Number

The number of molecules in one GMW of any substance is 6.02×10^{23}. This is shorthand for 602,000,000,000,000,000,000,000 molecules (See Appendix, *Exponents of 10*).

Talking about molecules in such astronomical numbers is incomprehensible. Therefore, Avogadro defined a GMW (also called a mole) as containing 6.02×10^{23} molecules.

Similarly, there are 6.02×10^{23} atoms in a GAW of any element.

In 1 GAW or 1 GEW of hydrogen there are 6.02×10^{23} ions.

In 1 GAW or 1 GEW of chloride there are 6.02×10^{23} ions.

Therefore:

$$6.02 \times 10^{23} \text{ ions of } H^+ + 6.02 \times 10^{23} \text{ ions of } Cl^-$$

$$\rightarrow 6.02 \times 10^{23} \text{ molecules of HCl}$$

However:

$$1 \text{ GEW } S^{--} + 1 \text{ GEW } H^+ \rightarrow 1 \text{ GEW } H_2S$$

$$\text{GEW of } S^{--} = \text{its GAW/valence} = 32 \text{ g}/2 = 16 \text{ g}$$

S^{--} has a valence of 2, so its GEW is half of its GAW. In other words, it takes 2 H^+ to "satisfy" 1 S^{--}.

$$16 \text{ g } S^{--} \text{ (or 1/2 GAW or 1 GEW)} + 1 \text{ g } H^+ \text{ (or 1 GAW or 1 GEW)}$$

$$\rightarrow 17 \text{ g } H_2S \text{ (or 1 GEW)}$$

How many ions and molecules does this equation represent?

one-half GAW (or 1 GEW) of S^{--}

is equal to one-half as many ions as 1 GAW.

6.02×10^{23} ions in 1 GAW $S^{--} \div 2$

$= 3.01 \times 10^{23}$ ions in 1 GEW S^{--}

Therefore, 3.01×10^{23} ions of S^{--} combine with 6.02×10^{23} ions of H^+ to make 3.01×10^{23} molecules of H_2S. (See Fig. 6.1.)

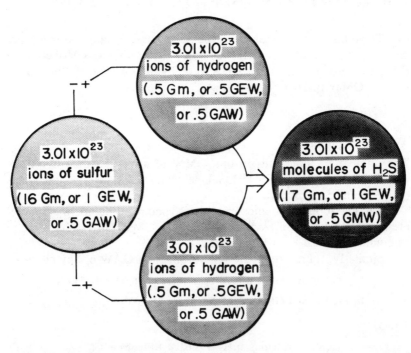

Figure 6.1. Diagram Showing How 3.01×10^{23} Ions of Sulfur Combine with 6.02×10^{23} Ions of Hydrogen to Make 3.01×10^{23} Molecules of H_2S

Figure 6.1 shows that only .5 GAW of S^{--} is needed to neutralize 1 GAW of H^+, because each S^{--} anion requires 2 H^+ cations to be "satisfied." After they combine, there are only 3.01×10^{23} molecules formed. This is 1 GEW, or .5 GMW, of H_2S.

GEW OF ACIDS, BASES, AND SALTS

GEW of Acids

The GEW of an acid molecule is equal to its GMW divided by the number of hydrogen ions in its formula. In the example just discussed, the GMW of H_2S is 34 g (because $1 + 1 + 32 = 34$). There are 2 H^+ in the formula. Therefore:

$$GEW \text{ of } H_2S = 34 \text{ g}/2 = 17 \text{ g}$$

The GEW of an acid is defined as the number of GMWs of the acid, or the fraction of 1 GMW of the acid, that contains 1 GAW of H^+. (Compare this statement with the definition of a GEW of an element or radical on page 71.)

Examples

$$GEW \text{ of an acid} = \frac{GMW \text{ of the acid}}{\text{number of } H^+ \text{ in the formula}}$$

$$GEW \text{ of } HCl = 36 \text{ g} \div 1 = 36 \text{ g}$$

$$GEW \text{ of } H_2SO_4 = 98 \text{ g} \div 2 = 49 \text{ g}$$

Important exceptions

When water ionizes, it does so only partially, i.e.,

$$H_2O \rightarrow H^+ + (OH)^-$$

The hydroxyl radical $(OH)^-$ is formed. All of the H^+ ions are not replaceable. One H^+ ion remains bound to the radical. Thus, the GEW of H_2O is equal to its GMW, rather than half of it, as might be expected, because there are 2 H^+ in its formula.

$$GEW \text{ of } H(OH) = 18 \div 1 = 18 \text{ g}$$

Another example of an extremely important electrolyte that ionizes partially is

$$H_2CO_3 \rightarrow H^+ + (HCO_3)^-$$

Here, too, one H^+ remains bound in the radical, which then behaves as a monovalent anion. (Monovalent means having a valence of 1.)

Therefore

$$\text{GEW of } H_2CO_3 = \frac{2 + 12 + 48 \text{ g}}{\text{valence of } 1} = 62 \text{ g/1} = 62 \text{ g}$$

GEW of Bases

The GEW of a base equals the number of GMWs of the base, or the fraction of 1 GMW of the base, that contains 1 GAW of $(OH)^-$.

$$\text{GEW of a base} = \frac{\text{GMW of the base}}{\text{number of } (OH)^- \text{ in its formula}}$$

$$\text{GEW of NaOH} = (23 + 16 + 1 \text{ g})/1 = 40 \text{ g/1} \qquad = 40 \text{ g}$$

$$\text{GEW of Ca(OH)}_2 = (40 + 16 + 1 + 16 + 1 \text{ g})/2 \qquad = 74 \text{ g/2} = 37 \text{ g}$$

Therefore, 37 g of $Ca(OH)_2$ contains 1 GAW of $(OH)^-$; 74 g of $Ca(OH)_2$ contains 2 GAW of $(OH)^-$.

GEW of Salts

$$\text{The GEW of a salt} = \frac{\text{GMW of the salt}}{\text{valence} \times \text{subscript}}$$

Most salts have no replaceable H^+ or $(OH)^-$ in their molecules, but all of them have a radical or ion with a positive valence that has combined with a radical or ion with a negative valence. So, if the number of cations (or + radicals) in the formula is multiplied by the valence of that cation (or radical), the number of + charges will be known.

Examples

$$\text{GEW of NaCl} = \frac{23 + 35 \text{ g}}{\text{valence of } 1 \times 1 \text{ ion of Na}^+} = 58 \text{ g}$$

$$\text{GEW of CaCl}_2 = \frac{40 + 35 + 35 \text{ g}}{\text{valence of } 2 \times 1 \text{ ion of Ca}^{++}} = \frac{110 \text{ Gm}}{2} = 55 \text{ g}$$

$$\text{GEW of Fe}_2O_3 = \frac{56 + 56 + 16 + 16 + 16 \text{ g}}{\text{valence of } 3 \times 2 \text{ ions of Fe}^{+++}} = \frac{160 \text{ g}}{6} = 26.6 \text{ g}$$

(This equation means that 26.6 g of Fe_2O_3 will react exactly with 1 GAW of hydrogen. This is only one-sixth of 1 GMW of Fe_2O_3.)

$$\text{GEW of NH}_4Cl = \frac{14 + 4 + 35 \text{ g}}{\text{valence of } 1 \times 1 \text{ ion of (NH}_4)^+} = 53 \text{ g}$$

MILLIEQUIVALENT WEIGHTS (mEq)

$$1,000 \text{ mEq} = 1 \text{ Eq}$$

just as

$$1,000 \text{ mg} = 1 \text{ g}$$

The milliequivalent, abbreviated mEq, equals .001 GEW, and is used for convenience as the unit of measure for electrolytes in biochemistry.

1 GEW of NaCl weighs 58 g

1 mEq of NaCl weighs 58 mg

1 GEW $CaCl_2$ weighs 55 g

1 mEq $CaCl_2$ weighs 55 mg

Chapter 7
WORKING WITH MILLIEQUIVALENTS

Chapter 6 explains that:

> 1 Eq of a cation + 1 Eq of an anion → 1 Eq of a compound

Therefore:

> 1 mEq of a cation + 1 mEq of an anion → 1 mEq of a compound

Example:

> 1 mEq H^+ + 1 mEq Cl^- → 1 mEq HCl

Since mEq and mg are the units of measure that are used in most laboratory reports and drug problems, they will be used in all problems and discussions that follow.

Interpreting laboratory reports depends on knowing that the sum of the mEq weights of all the compounds that react with each other in an equation (known as reactants) equals the sum of the mEq weights of all the compounds made as a result of the reaction (known as products). An example is:

1 mEq HCl (36 mg) + 1 mEq NaOH (40 mg)

> → 1 mEq HOH (18 mg) + 1 mEq NaCl (58 mg)

> 36 mg + 40 mg = 18 mg + 58 mg

> 76 mg = 76 mg

The equation is balanced.

The sum of the reactants equals the sum of the products, and every ion that exists in the reactants has been used to make the products. This fact will be more evident in the problems that follow.

Problem 1

How much HCl should be added to 20 mg of NaOH for an exact reaction to take place?

Step 1 Write the equation to see if it balances ion for ion, and radical for radical. Indicate the valence (charge) of each reactant, and each product.

$$Na^+(OH)^- + H^+Cl^- \rightarrow Na^+Cl^- + H^+(OH)^-$$

In the *reactants* there are: In the *products* there are:
    1 ion Na^+ 1 ion Na^+
    1 radical $(OH)^-$ 1 radical $(OH)^-$
    1 ion H^+ 1 ion H^+
    1 ion Cl^- 1 ion Cl^-

In this problem, there are the same number of ions and radicals in the products as there are in the reactants. Each ion and radical has its required number of "mates," which are all satisfied because all the reactants have a valence of 1.

Step 2   There are 20 mg of NaOH available. How many mEq is this? To answer this question, it is necessary to figure the mgMW of NaOH. Referring to Table 6.1:

	mg Atomic Weight
Na	23 mg
O	16 mg
H	1 mg
mgMW of NaOH	40 mg

Step 3   Determine the mEq weight of NaOH. The GEW or mgEW of a base is equal to mgMW of the base divided by the number of $(OH)^-$ in its formula. Therefore, the mEq weight of NaOH is:

$$\frac{40 \text{ mg}}{1} \text{ or } 40 \text{ mg/mEq}$$

In other words, there are 40 mg in each mEq of NaOH.

Step 4   Since 20 mg of NaOH are available, and 1 mEq of NaOH weighs 40 mg, the mEq of available NaOH is:

$$20 \text{ mg} \div 40 \text{ mg/mEq}$$

$$\overset{1}{\cancel{20 \text{ mg}}} \times \frac{\text{mEq}}{\underset{2}{\cancel{40 \text{ mg}}}} = 1/2 \text{ mEq or .5 mEq NaOH available}$$

Therefore, 20 mg NaOH is .5 mEq.

Step 5   Since:

$$1 \text{ mEq NaOH} + 1 \text{ mEq HCl} \rightarrow 1 \text{ mEq NaCl} + 1 \text{ mEq HOH}$$

Then:

$$.5 \text{ mEq NaOH} + .5 \text{ mEq HCl} \rightarrow .5 \text{ mEq NaCl} + .5 \text{ mEq HOH}$$

The weight of .5 mEq of each of the other compounds in the

equation must be calculated. Referring to Table 6.1:

HCl

	mgAW
H	1 mg
Cl	35 mg
mgMW of HCl	36 mg

$$\text{The mEq weight of an acid} = \frac{\text{mgMW of the acid}}{\text{number of } H^+ \text{ in the formula}}$$

Therefore, the mEq weight of HCl is 36 mg/1 or 36 mg/mEq. Since there are 36 mg in 1 mEq of HCl, there are 18 mg in .5 mEq of HCl.

NaCl

	mgAW
Na	23 mg
Cl	35 mg
mgMW of NaCl	58 mg

$$\text{The mEq weight of a salt} = \frac{\text{mgMW of the salt}}{\text{valence} \times \text{subscript}}$$

Therefore, the mEq weight of NaCl is 58 mg/(1 × 1) or 58 mg/mEq. Since there are 58 mg in each mEq of NaCl, there are 29 mg/.5 mEq NaCl.

HOH

	mgAW
H	1 mg
O	16 mg
H	1 mg
mgMW of HOH	18 mg

$$\text{The mEq weight of } H^+(OH)^- = \frac{\text{mgMW}}{\text{number of } H^+ \text{ in formula}}$$

$$= 18/1 = 18 \text{ mg/mEq}$$

There are 18 mg in each mEq of HOH, or 9 mg in .5 mEq of HOH.

　　Step 6　　.5 mEq NaOH (20 mg) + .5 mEq HCl (18 mg) → .5 mEq NaCl (29 mg) + .5 mEq HOH (9 mg).

$$20 \text{ mg} + 18 \text{ mg} = 29 \text{ mg} + 9 \text{ mg}$$

$$38 \text{ mg} = 38 \text{ mg}$$

　　The equation balances. Add 18 mg of HCl to the 20 mg of NaOH, and a complete, and exact reaction will occur. It will produce 29 mg of NaCl, and 9 mg of HOH.

Problem 2

The student should try to solve the following problem before referring to the discussion. How much NH_4OH will react exactly with 108 mg of HCl? $(NH_4)^+$ is a radical with a valence of $+1$.

Step 1 Write the equation to see that it balances, ion for ion and radical for radical. Indicate the valence of each reactant and each product.

$$(NH_4)^+(OH)^- + H^+Cl^- \rightarrow H^+(OH)^- + (NH_4)^+Cl^-$$

In the *reactants* there are:
   1 radical $(NH_4)^+$
   1 radical $(OH)^-$
   1 ion H^+
   1 ion Cl^-

In the *products* there are:
   1 radical $(NH_4)^+$
   1 radical $(OH)^-$
   1 ion H^+
   1 ion Cl^-

There are the same number of ions and radicals in the products as there are in the reactants. Each ion and radical has the required number of "mates." All of the reactants have a valence of 1. Therefore, the equation balances.

Step 2 There are 108 mg of HCl available. How many mEq are there in 108 mg of HCl?

Figure the mgMW of HCL, as in problem 1. The mgMW of HCl is 36 mg. Problem 1 also illustrates that the mEq weight of HCl is 36 mg. Since there are 36 mg in each mEq of HCl:

$$108 \text{ mg HCl} \div 36 \text{ mg/mEq} = \overset{3}{\cancel{108 \text{ mg}}} \times \frac{\text{mEq}}{\cancel{36 \text{ mg}}} = 3 \text{ mEq of HCl}$$

Step 3 Since 3 mEq of HCl are available, the weight of 3 mEq of each of the other compounds in the equation must be figured. The equation should look like this:

$$3 \text{ mEq HCl} + 3 \text{ mEq NH}_4\text{OH} \rightarrow 3 \text{ mEq NH}_4\text{Cl} + 3 \text{ mEq HOH}$$

NH₄OH

	mgAW
N	14 mg
4 atoms of H	4 mg
O	16 mg
H	1 mg
mgMW of NH_4OH	35 mg

$$\text{mEq weight of a base} = \frac{\text{mgMW of the base}}{\text{number of (OH)}^- \text{ in formula}}$$

$$\text{mEq weight of NH}_4\text{OH} = 35 \text{ mg/1} = 35 \text{ mg/mEq}$$

There are 35 mg in each mEq of NH_4OH, and there are 105 mg in 3 mEq NH_4OH.

NH_4Cl

	mgAW
N	14 mg
4 atoms of H	4 mg
Cl	35 mg
mgMW of NH_4Cl	53 mg

$$\text{mEq weight of a salt} = \frac{\text{mgMW of the salt}}{\text{valence} \times \text{subscript}}$$

$$\text{mEq weight of } NH_4Cl = 53 \text{ mg}/(1 \times 1) = 53 \text{ mg/mEq}$$

There are 53 mg in each mEq of NH_4Cl, and there are 159 mg in 3 mEq NH_4Cl.

HOH

Problem 1 shows that there are 18 mg/mEq of HOH.

Since there are 18 mg in each mEq of HOH,

there are 54 mg in 3 mEq of HOH.

Step 4   Write the final equation:

$$3 \text{ mEq } NH_4OH \ (105 \text{ mg}) + 3 \text{ mEq HCl } (108 \text{ mg})$$

$$\rightarrow 3 \text{ mEq } NH_4Cl \ (159 \text{ mg}) + 3 \text{ mEq HOH } (54 \text{ mg})$$

$$105 \text{ mg} + 108 \text{ mg} = 159 \text{ mg} + 54 \text{ mg}$$

$$213 \text{ mg} = 213 \text{ mg}$$

The equation balances. Add 105 mg of NH_4OH to the 108 mg of HCl, and a complete, and exact reaction will occur, which will produce 159 mg of NH_4Cl and 54 mg of HOH.

Problem 3

This problem involves determining valence. How much NaOH will react exactly with 147 mg of H_2SO_4?

Step 1   Write the equation to see if it balances, ion for ion and radical for radical. Indicate the valence of each compound.

$$H_2{}^+(SO_4)^{--} + Na^+(OH)^- \rightarrow Na^+(SO_4)^{--} + H^+(OH)^-$$

In the *reactants* there are:
2 ions H^+
1 radical $(SO_4)^{--}$
1 ion Na^+
1 radical $(OH)^-$

In the *products* there are:
1 ion H^+
1 radical $(SO_4)^{--}$
1 ion Na^+
1 radical $(OH)^-$

This equation does not balance.

1. What happened to the other ion of H^+ in the product?
2. "Bigamist" $(SO_4)^{--}$ has only 1 "mate" in the product.

To rectify this situation, notice in the product that $(SO_4)^{--}$ would be satisfied if there were 2 Na^+ ions to react with it. Make the compound in the product $Na_2^+(SO_4)^{--}$. If this is done, there must be 2 NaOH in the reactants, so that 2 Na^+ ions are available to combine with the $(SO_4)^{--}$ in the product. The equation now looks like this:

$$H_2^+(SO_4)^{--} + 2\,Na^+(OH)^- \rightarrow Na_2^+(SO_4)^{--} + H^+(OH)^-$$

The number of Na^+ ions and $(SO_4)^{--}$ radicals balance. But the $(OH)^-$ radical added with the second Na^+ still needs to be used, and there is an extra H^+ that is unaccounted for. Combine the H^+ and the $(OH)^-$ and add it to the HOH already in the equation. Now the equation balances:

$$H_2^+(SO_4)^{--} + 2\,Na^+(OH)^- \rightarrow Na_2^+(SO_4)^{--} + 2\,H^+(OH)^-$$

In the *reactants*, there are:	In the *products*, there are:
2 ions H^+	2 ions H^+
1 radical $(SO_4)^{--}$	1 radical $(SO_4)^{--}$
2 ions Na^+	2 ions Na^+
2 radicals $(OH)^-$	2 radicals $(OH)^-$

All ions and radicals in the reactants have been used in the products and all "bigamists" have been satisfied. The equation balances.

A lot of this juggling can be eliminated by the use of mEq from the beginning omitting step 1 entirely. This is the beauty of the equivalent system. All that must be done is to see that the "bigamists" are satisfied, using mEq as shown in steps 2 & 3, below.

Step 2   There are 147 mg of H_2SO_4 available. How many mEq are there in 147 mg of H_2SO_4? Figure the mgMW of H_2SO_4.

	mgAW
2 atoms H	2 mg
S	32 mg
4 atoms O	64 mg
mgMW H_2SO_4	98 mg

$$\text{mEq weight of an acid} = \frac{\text{mgMW of the acid}}{\text{number of } H^+ \text{ in the formula}}$$

mEq weight of H_2SO_4 = 98 mg/2 = 49 mg/mEq

Since there are 147 mg of H_2SO_4:

$$147\ mg \div 49\ mg/mEq = \overset{3}{\cancel{147\ mg}} \times \frac{mEq}{\cancel{49\ mg}} = 3\ mEq\ of\ H_2SO_4$$

Step 3   Since 3 mEq of H_2SO_4 are available, the weight of 3 mEq of each of the other compounds in the equation must be calculated, so the following equation is used:

$$3 \text{ mEq } H_2SO_4 + 3 \text{ mEq NaOH} \rightarrow 3 \text{ mEq } Na_2SO_4 + 3 \text{ mEq HOH}$$

NaOH

Calculate the mgMW of NaOH as done in problem 1.

The mgMW of NaOH is 40 mg.

The mEq weight of NaOH was also shown to be 40 mg/mEq.

Since there are 40 mg/mEq of NaOH,

there are 120 mg in 3 mEq of NaOH.

Na_2SO_4

Calculate the mgMW of Na_2SO_4.

	mgAW
2 atoms Na	46 mg
S	32 mg
4 atoms O	64 mg
mgMW of Na_2SO_4	142 mg

$$\text{mEq weight of a salt} = \frac{\text{mgMW of the salt}}{\text{valence} \times \text{subscript}}$$

$$\text{mEq weight of } Na_2SO_4 = 142 \text{ mg}/(1 \times 2) = 71 \text{ mg/mEq}$$

Since there are 71 mg in each mEq of Na_2SO_4, there are 213 mg in 3 mEq of Na_2SO_4.

HOH

Calculate the mgMW of HOH, as illustrated in problem 1.

Both the mgMW and the mEq weight of HOH equal 18 mg.

Since there are 18 mg in 1 mEq of HOH,

there are 54 mg in 3 mEq of HOH.

Step 4   Write the final equation:

$$3 \text{ mEq } H_2SO_4 \text{ (147 mg)} + 3 \text{ mEq NaOH (120 mg)}$$

$$\rightarrow 3 \text{ mEq } Na_2SO_4 \text{ (213 mg)} + 3 \text{ mEq HOH (54 mg)}$$

$$147 \text{ mg} + 120 \text{ mg} = 213 \text{ mg} + 54 \text{ mg}$$

$$267 \text{ mg} = 267 \text{ mg}$$

The equation balances. Add 120 mg of NaOH to 147 mg of H_2SO_4, and a complete and exact reaction will occur. The products will be 213 mg of Na_2SO_4 and 54 mg of HOH.

Chapter 8
CLINICAL LABORATORY REPORTS

If the slip accompanying a patient's blood sample requests the amount of sodium that is present in the plasma, the sample could be analyzed for plasma sodium content in mg%. However, the number of mg of sodium in 100 ml of plasma would mean little to the doctor who needs to know *exactly* how the patient's body is maintaining its electrolyte balance right now. The doctor needs to know the number of sodium ions that exist in each liter of plasma in order to treat the patient intelligently. Therefore, the sodium content of the blood plasma is measured in mEq/L.

Sodium is the major cation that exists in the blood plasma. Table 8.1 lists the concentration of normal plasma electrolytes. If a patient's laboratory report indicates that his sodium concentration falls outside the normal range of 135–155 mEq/L of plasma, the patient has a sodium imbalance which should be corrected.

Total electrolyte concentration in the plasma is equal to 154 mEq cations/L, and 154 mEq anions/L. The total cations always equal the total anions. They balance each other. (See definition of homeostasis, Chap. 5, p. 63.) This equality would not be apparent if the concentration of the various electrolytes were expressed in mg%. It must be remembered that mEq deal with the number of ions, not their weights. The advantages of the mEq expression are:

1. Calculations are greatly simplified for the doctor who needs to treat the patient for electrolyte imbalances.
2. Electrolyte imbalances are much easier to evaluate at a glance.
3. Electrolyte shifts are impossible to follow unless they are expressed as mEq/L. In other words, when there is a deficit in one cation, another cation may increase, or, if there is an excess in one anion, another anion may decrease, or there may be a deficit or excess of both cations and anions. Electrolytes in the body can shift in many different ways because the law of nature requiring that cations must always equal anions sometimes interferes with

Table 8.1   Normal Plasma Electrolytes

Cations	mEq/L	Normal Lab Range (mEq/L)	Anions	mEq/L	Normal Lab Range (mEq/L)
Na$^+$	142	135–155	(HCO$_3$)$^-$	24	23–28
K$^+$	5	3.6–5.5	Cl$^-$	105	98–109
Ca^{++}	5	4.5–5.7	(HPO$_4$)$^{--}$	2	
Mg^{++}	2	1.5–2.4	(SO$_4$)$^{--}$	1	
			(Organic Acid)$^-$	6	
			(Proteinate)$^-$	16	
	$\overline{154}$ mEq/L			$\overline{154}$ mEq/L	

the body's attempt to keep each individual electrolyte within the normal, healthy range listed in Table 8.1. The plasma electrolyte report from the laboratory shows the patient's electrolyte status at the particular moment that the blood specimen was drawn. Sometimes it indicates a serious or life-threatening electrolyte imbalance. When it does, the doctor is guided by this report to adjust fluid and electrolyte intake and output with diet and drugs. In this way the body is assisted to overcome the illness that is causing the electrolyte imbalance. In addition, the doctor may order specific electrolytes to be given orally, or by intravenous infusion, if necessary.

Problems

Modern laboratory computer-like machines report most electrolytes in mEq/L of plasma. In order to understand the significance of mEq weights, a few problems of conversion of laboratory reports from mg% to mEq/L will be included here.

Problem 1

Convert 322 mg% of sodium to mEq/L.

Step 1   Table 6.1 shows that the GAW of Na$^+$ is 23 g (or the mgAW is 23 mg). Na$^+$ is monovalent, so its mEq weight is also 23 mg.

Step 2   The specimen contains Na$^+$ 322 mg%, or 322 mg/100 ml of blood plasma. Since sodium content is expressed in mEq/L of plasma, 322 mg% is multiplied by 10 to get mg/L of plasma.

$$\text{plasma Na}^+ = \frac{322 \text{ mg} \times 10}{100 \text{ ml} \times 10} = \frac{3,220 \text{ mg}}{1,000 \text{ ml}} = 3,220 \text{ mg/L}$$

Step 3 In 1 mEq of Na$^+$, there are 23 mg, expressed as 23 mg/mEq.

$$\text{mEq of Na}^+ = 3,220 \text{ mg/L} \div 23 \text{ mg/mEq}$$

$$= \frac{\overset{140}{\cancel{3,220} \text{ mg}}}{L} \times \frac{\text{mEq}}{\cancel{23} \text{ mg}} = 140 \text{ mEq/L of plasma}$$

Step 4 The answer 140 mEq/L is compared with the normal plasma electrolyte concentrations listed in Table 8.1. How far and in what direction the patient's sodium concentration deviates from the normal range is noted. This patient's laboratory report is well within the normal range.

Problem 2

Convert 350 mg% of Na$^+$ to mEq/L.

Step 1 The mgAW of Na$^+$ is 23 mg. The mEq weight of Na$^+$ is also 23 mg.

Step 2

$$\text{plasma Na}^+ = \frac{350 \text{ mg} \times 10 = 3,500 \text{ mg}}{100 \text{ ml} \times 10 = 1,000 \text{ ml}} \text{ , or } 3,500 \text{ mg/L}$$

Step 3

$$\text{plasma Na}^+ = 3,500 \text{ mg/L} \div 23 \text{ mg/mEq} = \frac{\overset{152}{\cancel{3,500} \text{ mg}}}{L} \times \frac{\text{mEq}}{\cancel{23} \text{ mg}} = 152 \text{ mEq/L}$$

Step 4 Compared with the table of normal concentrations in Table 8.1, it is noted that this plasma Na$^+$ is in the high-normal range.

Problem 3

Convert 19.5 mg% of plasma K$^+$ to mEq/L.

Step 1 The mgAW of K$^+$ is 39 mg. Since K$^+$ is monovalent, the mEq weight is also 39 mg.

Step 2

$$\text{plasma K}^+ = \frac{19.5 \text{ mg} \times 10 = 195 \text{ mg}}{100 \text{ ml} \times 10 = 1,000 \text{ ml}} \text{ , or } 195 \text{ mg/L}$$

Step 3

$$195 \text{ mg/L} \div 39 \text{ mg/mEq} = \frac{\overset{5}{\cancel{195} \text{ mg}}}{L} \times \frac{\text{mEq}}{\cancel{39} \text{ mg}} = 5 \text{ mEq/L of plasma}$$

Step 4 Compared with K^+ normal concentrations in Table 8.1, this patient's plasma K^+ is in the high-normal range.

Problem 4

Convert 40 mg% of plasma K^+ to mEq/L.

Step 1   The mgAW of K^+ is 39 mg. Since K^+ is monovalent, the mEq weight is also 39 mg.

Step 2

$$\text{plasma } K^+ = \frac{40 \text{ mg}}{100 \text{ ml}} \times \frac{10}{10} = \frac{400 \text{ mg}}{1{,}000 \text{ ml}} = 400 \text{ mg/L}$$

Step 3

$$400 \text{ mg/L} \div 39 \text{ mg/mEq} = \frac{\overset{10.2}{\cancel{400 \text{ mg}}}}{L} \times \frac{\text{mEq}}{\cancel{39 \text{ mg}}} = 10.2 \text{ mEq/L of plasma}$$

Step 4 Compared with the normal concentrations in Table 8.1, this patient's plasma K^+ concentration is dangerously high, a fact which requires immediate treatment.

Problem 5

Convert 20 mg% of plasma Ca^{++} to mEq/L.

Step 1

$$\text{mgAW of } Ca^{++} = 40 \text{ mg}$$

Ca^{++} is bivalent, i.e., it requires two "mates." One H^+ ion can be replaced by only half a Ca^{++} ion, or 1 Ca^{++} ion can replace 2 H^+ ions. By definition:

mEq weight of Ca^{++} = 40 mg/2 or 20 mg/mEq   (Review Chap. 6.)

Step 2

$$\text{plasma } Ca^{++} = \frac{20 \text{ mg}}{100 \text{ ml}} \times \frac{10}{10} = \frac{200 \text{ mg}}{1{,}000 \text{ ml}} \text{ or } 200 \text{ mg/L}$$

Step 3

$$\text{plasma } Ca^{++} = 200 \text{ mg/L} \div 20 \text{ mg/mEq} = \frac{\overset{10}{\cancel{200 \text{ mg}}}}{L} \times \frac{\text{mEq}}{\cancel{20 \text{ mg}}} = 10 \text{ mEq/L}$$

Step 4 Compared with the normal concentrations in Table 8.1, this patient's plasma Ca^{++} concentration is high.

Problem 6

Explain why:

$$23 \text{ mg of } Na^+ = 20 \text{ mg of } Ca^{++}$$

The atomic weight of Na^+ is 23 mg, and of Ca^{++} is 40 mg; 1 mEq of Na^+ weighs 23 mg and 1 mEq of Ca^{++} weighs 40/2 or 20 mg.

The equality, 23 mg Na^+ = 20 mg Ca^{++}, is one way of expressing that 1 mEq of Na^+ has the same combining power as 1 mEq of Ca^{++}. It means that either 23 mg of Na^+ or 20 mg of Ca^{++} can replace 1 mg of H^+.

To further illustrate the significance of this equality, recall that 1 mEq of a cation exactly balances 1 mEq of an anion.

1 mEq Na^+ (23 mg) + 1 mEq Cl^- (35 mg) → 1 mEq NaCl (58 mg)

   Proof: 23 mg + 35 mg = 58 mg

1 mEq Ca^{++} (20 mg) + 1 mEq Cl^- (35 mg) → 1 mEq $CaCl_2$ (55 mg)

   Proof: 20 mg + 35 mg = (40 mg + 35 mg + 35 mg)/2 = 55 mg

These two equations illustrate how 35 mg of chloride combine with a monovalent and a bivalent cation. The 35 mg of Cl^- combines with 1 Na^+ ion, but satisfies only 1/2 Ca^{++} ion.

It should now be understood why 1 Cl^- ion, a monovalent anion weighing 35 mg, is as effective in balancing the charge on any monovalent cation, such as H^+ weighing only 1 mg, as is a monovalent anion such as albuminate that weighs in excess of 68,000 mg. The equations below illustrate this point:

$$1 \text{ mg } H^+ + 35 \text{ mg } Cl^- \rightarrow 36 \text{ mg HCl}$$

$$1 \text{ mEq } H^+ + 1 \text{ mEq } Cl^- \rightarrow 1 \text{ mEq HCl}$$

$$1 \text{ mg } H^+ + 68,000 \text{ mg albuminate}^- \rightarrow 68,001 \text{ mg albumin}$$

$$1 \text{ mEq } H^+ + 1 \text{ mEq albuminate}^- \rightarrow 1 \text{ mEq albumin}$$

$$1 \text{ mg } H^+ + 17 \text{ mg } (OH)^- \rightarrow 18 \text{ mg HOH (water)}$$

$$1 \text{ mEq } H^+ + 1 \text{ mEq } (OH)^- \rightarrow 1 \text{ mEq HOH}$$

SUMMARY

1. The mEq system is a way to measure body concentrations of specific ions, known as electrolytes.
2. In the body there is an optimum concentration of each electrolyte in each tissue or fluid compartment.
3. The laboratory technician measures the concentration of the various electrolytes in the specimen received and reports them in a manner that the doctor can evaluate at a glance.
4. The kidneys and lungs strive to maintain an optimum state of each electrolyte in the body. These two organs prevent the loss or

retention of each specific ion, according to its plasma concentration, on a minute-to-minute basis.

5.   Total cation concentration is an index to total electrolyte concentration, since the number of cations equals the number of anions. Cations are not interchangeable in the body. If one cation is depleted, a shift occurs to maintain electrical balance, but this occurrence is quickly apparent because the patient gets sick. The anions may shift to a greater extent before the patient is obviously sick.

REVIEW

The following statements should make sense. If they do not, a review of all the material in this section is necessary.

1.   An equivalent weight is a combining weight. Therefore, since 1 mEq of Ca^{++} weighs 20 mg, 20 mg of Ca^{++} will replace 1 mEq (1 mg) of H^+, or will combine with 1 mEq of any anion.

2.   mEq weight = mg atomic weight/valence

3.   mEq weight of Ca^{++} = 40 mg/2 = 20 mg

4.   1 mEq Cl^- weighs 35 mg

5.   1 mEq H^+ weighs 1 mg

6.   1 mEq Fe^{+++} weighs 56 mg/3 or 18.6 mg

7.   1 mEq O^{--} weighs 16 mg/2 or 8 mg

8.   1 mEq K^+ weighs 39 mg

9.   1 mEq Na^+ weighs 23 mg

10. 1 mEq S^{--} weighs 32 mg/2 or 16 mg

11. 1 mEq $(HCO_3)^-$ weighs (1 + 12 + 16 + 16 + 16 mg) or 61 mg

12. 1 mEq $(OH)^-$ weighs (16 + 1 mg) or 17 mg

13. 1 mEq $(SO_4)^{--}$ weighs (32 + 16 + 16 + 16 + 16 mg)/2 or 48 mg

14. 1 mEq Ca^{++} weighs 40 mg/2 or 20 mg = 1 mEq Na^+ weighs 23 mg/1 or 23 mg

15. 1 mEq weight of Na^+ (23 mg) = 1 mEq weight of Ca^{++} (20 mg)

16. 1 mEq S^{--} (which weighs 16 mg) = 1 mEq $(SO_4)^{--}$ (which weighs 48 mg)

17. 1 mEq Na^+ (which weighs 23 mg) = 1 mEq H^+ (which weighs 1 mg)

18. 1 mEq S^{--} (which weighs 16 mg) = 1 mEq $(OH)^-$ (which weighs 17 mg)

19. 1 mgAW of Ca^{++} (which weighs 40 mg) + 2 mgAW of Cl^- (which weigh 70 mg) = 1 mgMW $CaCl_2$ (which weighs 110 mg)

20. 1 mEq Ca^{++} (which weighs 20 mg) + 1 mEq Cl^- (which weighs 35 mg) = 1 mEq $CaCl_2$ (which weighs 55 mg)

21. 1 mEq weight of $CaCl_2$ = mgMW/valence = (40 + 35 + 35 mg)/ 2 = 55 mg
(Notice that problems 20 and 21 are identical. Number 21 figures the mEq weight directly from the molecule $CaCl_2$.)

22. 2 mgAW H^+ (which weigh 2 mg) + 1 mgAW $(SO_4)^{--}$ (which weighs 32 + 64 mg or 96 mg) = 1 mgMW H_2SO_4 (which weighs 2 + 32 + 64 or 98 mg)

23. 1 mEq H^+ (which weighs 1 mg) + 1 mEq $(SO_4)^{--}$ (which weighs 48 mg) = 1 mEq H_2SO_4 (which weighs 49 mg)

24. mEq weight of H_2SO_4 = $\dfrac{\text{mg MW}}{\text{number of } H^+ \text{ in formula}}$ = (2 + 32 + 64 mg)/2 = 49 mg
(Notice that problems 23 and 24 are identical. Problem 24 figures the mEq weight directly from the molecule H_2SO_4.)

REVIEW PROBLEMS

Brief answers for these review problems follow without explanation.

1. Name two biochemical factors that are significant in homeostasis of living bodies.
2. Define an electrolyte.
3. Differentiate between strong and weak electrolytes.
4. Define an equivalent weight.
5. What does an equivalent weight measure?
6. What is a milliequivalent weight?
7. What is the GEW of an element? of a radical?
8. 1 GAW Cl^- + 1 GAW H^+ → 1 GMW HCl
What is the GEW of the Cl^-?
9. 1 GAW S^{--} + 2 GAW H^+ → 1 GMW H_2S
What is the GEW of the S^{--}?
10. What is the formula for a GEW of an element or radical?
11. Define valence.
12. How is the GEW of an acid determined? of a base? of a salt?
13. What is an important exception to the rule for figuring the mEq weight of an acid?
14. mgEW (or mEq weight) of Fe_2O_3 = 160/6 or 26.6 mg. What does the 26.6 mg represent?
15. Prove that HCl + NaOH → HOH + NaCl
16. If 60 mg of NaOH are available, how much HCl is needed for an exact reaction?
17. If 72 mg of HCl are available, how much NH_4OH will make an exact reaction?

18. If 24.5 mg of H_2SO_4 are available, how much NaOH will make an exact reaction?
19. If the number of mg of an electrolyte is known, how can the number of mEq be calculated?
20. If a laboratory report of an electrolyte is given in mg%, how can the mEq/L be determined?
21. How many mEq are there in 220 mg of $CaCl_2$?

Answers to Review Problems

1. Electrical balance or neutrality. The number of cations equals the number of anions. The body strives to keep the specific normal concentration of each cation and each anion at all times.
2. An electrolyte is any substance in an aqueous solution that can carry an electric current. Molecules split or dissociate into + or − ions.
3. Inorganic compounds such as HCl, NaOH, or NaCl are strong electrolytes and dissociate almost completely in water to + and − ions. They are excellent conductors of electricity.
    Organic electrolyte compounds are poor conductors of electricity. They dissociate only partially in water, and many of their molecules remain in the molecular form.
4. An equivalent is the chemical combining ability of an element equivalent to the combining ability of 1 GAW of H^+.
5. An equivalent weight measures the number of charges on an ion, (not its gram weight).
6. A milliequivalent weight equals .001 of an equivalent weight.
7. The GEW of an element (or a radical) is the number of GAWs, or the fraction of its GAW that can combine with or replace 1 GAW of H^+.
8. The GEW of Cl^- is 35 g.
9. The GEW of S^{--} is 16 g.
10. The GEW of an element or radical is its GAW/valence.
11. Valence is the number of ions of hydrogen which one anion of an element can hold in combination, or the number of ions of hydrogen that one cation of another element can displace.
12. $$\text{GEW of an acid} = \frac{\text{GMW of the acid}}{\text{number of } H^+ \text{ in the formula}}$$
    $$\text{GEW of a base} = \frac{\text{GMW of the base}}{\text{number of } (OH)^- \text{ in the formula}}$$
    $$\text{GEW of a salt} = \frac{\text{GMW of the salt}}{\text{valence} \times \text{subscript}}$$
13. H_2CO_3 is a weak organic acid that dissociates to $H^+ + (HCO_3)^-$.

14. For an exact reaction to take place 26.6 mg of Fe_2O_3 is required to replace 1 mg (1 mEq) of H^+.

15. 1 mEq HCl + 1 mEq NaOH $\rightarrow$ 1 mEq HOH + 1 mEq NaCl
     $$(1 + 35 \text{ mg}) + (23 + 16 + 1 \text{ mg}) = (1 + 16 + 1 \text{ mg}) + (23 + 35 \text{ mg})$$
     $$36 \text{ mg} + 40 \text{ mg} = 18 \text{ mg} + 58 \text{ mg}$$
     $$76 \text{ mg} = 76 \text{ mg}$$

16. To react exactly with 60 mg of NaOH, 1.5 mEq or 54 mg of HCl is needed.

17. To react exactly with 72 mg of HCl, 2 mEq or 70 mg of NH_4OH is needed.

18. To react exactly with 24.5 mg of H_2SO_4, .5 mEq or 20 mg of NaOH is needed.

19. $$mEq = \frac{\text{mg of the electrolyte available}}{\text{mEq weight of the electrolyte}}$$
     Example: If 105 mg of Cl^- are available, the number of mEq is 105/35 which equals 3 mEq.

20. mEq/L = (mg% $\times$ 10)/mEq weight
     Example: Na^+ = 322 mg%
     $$mEq/L \text{ of } Na^+ = (322 \times 10)/23 = 140 \text{ mEq/L}$$

21. 4 mEq

Chapter 9
PROBLEMS INVOLVING DOSAGES OF ELECTROLYTE DRUGS

Some electrolyte drugs are manufactured as powders, tablets, or capsules designed for oral or topical use, but of most concern are those made for intravenous injection. Some examples of such drugs are Sodium bicarbonate ($NaHCO_3$), 50-ml ampoules; Potassium chloride (KCl), 10-ml ampoules; Calcium chloride ($CaCl_2$), 10-ml ampoules; and Ringer's lactate, 1-L or 500-ml bottles.

Perhaps it is necessary to give a patient bicarbonate or calcium or potassium. Unfortunately there is no way to give the desired ion without its "mate." K^+ cannot be given without its Cl^- (or other anion); $(HCO_3)^-$ cannot be given without its Na^+, for example. Sometimes this can be an important factor in the treatment of a patient, if, for example, the patient needs bicarbonate, but should not have any sodium.

Problem 1

The label on a sodium bicarbonate ampoule specifies its contents:

"Sodium bicarbonate 50-ml size

$NaHCO_3$ 75 mg/ml

50 ml = 44.6 mEq"

Exactly how much sodium does the ampoule contain? Prove that the label is correct.

The exact *number* of $(HCO_3)^-$ ions and Na^+ ions that are in the 50-ml ampoule must be known before a decision can be made concerning the dosage required by the patient. He may need a whole ampoule, part of an ampoule, or several ampoules. Current plasma electrolyte and blood gas reports should be available to help in making this decision. The number of mEq of $NaHCO_3$ in this 50-ml ampoule must be known.

Step 1

$$\text{total mEq in the ampoule} = \frac{\text{mg available}}{\text{mEq weight of the compound}}$$

Calculate the weight of 1 mEq of $NaHCO_3$ from Table 6.1:

$$\text{mgAW of } Na^+ = 23 \text{ mg}$$

$$\text{mgAW of } (HCO_3)^- = (1 + 12 + 48 \text{ mg}) = 61 \text{ mg}$$

$$\text{mgMW of } NaHCO_3 = (23 + 61 \text{ mg}) = 84 \text{ mg}$$

Both Na^+ and $(HCO_3)^-$ are monovalent, so their mgAWs equal their mEq weights.

$$\text{mEq weight of a salt} = \frac{\text{mgMW}}{\text{valence} \times \text{subscript}}$$

$$\text{mEq weight of } NaHCO_3 = 84 \text{ mg}/(1 \times 1) = 84 \text{ mg/mEq}$$

Step 2   There are 84 mg in each mEq of $NaHCO_3$. How many mEq are there in the entire 50-ml ampoule? Since there are 75 mg/ml, there are:

$$\frac{75 \text{ mg}}{\text{ml}} \times 50 \text{ ml} = 3750 \text{ mg } NaHCO_3 \text{ in the entire 50-ml ampoule.}$$

Step 3

$$\text{total mEq in the ampoule} = \frac{\text{mg available}}{\text{mEq weight of the compound}}$$

$$\text{mEq } NaHCO_3 \text{ in this 50-ml ampoule} = \frac{3750 \text{ mg}}{84 \text{ mg/mEq}}$$

$$3750 \text{ mg} \div \frac{84 \text{ mg}}{\text{mEq}} = \overset{44.6}{\cancel{3750} \text{ mg}} \times \frac{\text{mEq}}{\cancel{84 \text{ mg}}}$$

$$= 44.6 \text{ mEq of } NaHCO_3$$

Step 4   If the patient is given the entire ampoule, he will have received:

$$44.6 \text{ mEq of } Na^+ + 44.6 \text{ mEq of } (HCO_3)^- = 44.6 \text{ mEq of } NaHCO_3$$

The patient will have received 44.6 mEq of sodium. The label is correct.

Problem 2

A common ampoule found on intensive care wards is potassium chloride. The label on the KCl ampoule specifies its contents thus:

"Potassium chloride   KCl

149 mg/ml   2 mEq/ml

10-ml size"

Prove that the label is correct. Calculate the number of mEq of KCl contained in the entire ampoule.

Step 1

$$\text{total mEq in the ampoule} = 2 \text{ mEq/} \cancel{ml} \times 10 \cancel{ml} = 20 \text{ mEq}$$

To calculate total mEq from total mg available:

$$149 \text{ mg/ml} \times 10 \text{ ml} = 1490 \text{ mg of KCl in the entire 10-ml ampoule}$$

$$\text{total mEq} = \frac{\text{total mg available}}{\text{mEq weight of the compound}}$$

from Table 6.1:

$$\text{mgAW K}^+ = 39 \text{ mg}$$

$$\text{mgAW Cl}^- = 35 \text{ mg}$$

$$\text{mgMW KCl} = 74 \text{ mg}$$

$$\text{mEq weight of KCl} = \frac{\text{mgMW}}{\text{valence} \times \text{subscript}} = 74 \text{ mg/}(1 \times 1) = 74 \text{ mg/mEq}$$

Step 2   Since there are 1490 mg of KCl in the ampoule, and there are 74 mg in each mEq of KCl:

$$\text{mEq of KCl in this 10-ml ampoule} = 1490 \text{ mg} \div 74 \text{ mg/mEq}$$

$$= \overset{20}{\cancel{1490 \text{ mg}}} \times \frac{\text{mEq}}{\cancel{74 \text{ mg}}} = 20 \text{ mEq of KCl}$$

Step 3   The label is correct. The ampoule contains:

$$20 \text{ mEq of K}^+ + 20 \text{ mEq of Cl}^- \text{ or } 20 \text{ mEq of KCl}$$

Problem 3

A 10-ml ampoule of calcium chloride is labeled thus:

"Calcium chloride $CaCl_2$ 10 ml = 1 g"

How many mEq of Ca^{++} are there in this ampoule?

Step 1

$$\text{total mEq in the ampoule} = \frac{\text{mg available}}{\text{mEq weight of the compound}}$$

Calculate the mEq weight of 1 mEq of $CaCl_2$ from Table 6.1:

$$\text{mgAW of Ca}^{++} = 40 \text{ mg}$$

$$\text{mgAW of Cl}^- = 35 \text{ mg}$$

$$\text{mEq weight of a salt} = \frac{\text{mgMW}}{\text{valence} \times \text{subscript}}$$

$$\text{mEq weight of CaCl}_2 = (40 \text{ mg} + 70 \text{ mg})/(2 \times 1)$$

$$= 110 \text{ mg/2} = 55 \text{ mg/mEq}$$

Step 2   Since there is 1 g or 1,000 mg of $CaCl_2$ in the 10-ml ampoule and there are 55 mg/mEq of $CaCl_2$:

mEq of $CaCl_2$ in this 10-ml ampoule = 1,000 mg ÷ 55 mg/mEq

$$= \overset{18.1}{\cancel{1,000\,mg}} \times \frac{mEq}{\cancel{55\,mg}}$$

$$= 18.1 \text{ mEq } CaCl_2$$

Step 3   There are 18.1 mEq of Ca^{++} in the entire ampoule.

18.1 mEq of Ca^{++} + 18.1 mEq Cl^- = 18.1 mEq of $CaCl_2$

Problem 4

The label on another calcium ampoule reads:

"Calcium gluceptate   5 ml

Each 5 ml = .09 g calcium"

How many mEq of Ca^{++} are in this ampoule?

Step 1   The formula for gluceptate is not known. The mEq weight of Ca^{++} is 20 mg/mEq.

Step 2   .09 g of calcium = 90 mg total amount of Ca^{++} in the 5-ml ampoule

Step 3

mEq of Ca^{++} in this ampoule = 90 mg ÷ 20 mg/mEq

$$= \overset{4.5}{\cancel{90\,mg}} \times \frac{mEq}{\cancel{20\,mg}} = 4.5 \text{ mEq}$$

4.5 mEq of Ca^{++} + 4.5 mEq of gluceptate$^-$ = 4.5 mEq of calcium gluceptate

There are 4.5 mEq of Ca^{++} in the ampoule.

Problem 5

A good examination problem would be to prove the label on a 1,000-ml bottle of Ringer's lactate. Prove that the number of mg of each electrolyte does, in fact, equal the number of mEq of each electrolyte as listed on the label. Figure the number of mEq there are of each ion, and then add them to see if the total mEq of cations equals the total mEq of anions.

A 1,000-ml bottle of Ringer's lactate is labeled thus:

Ringer's Lactate

1,000-ml size

Each 100 ml contains:		Each 1,000 ml contains:			
		Cations:		Anions:	
NaCl	600 mg	Na^+	130 mEq	Cl^-	109 mEq
Na Lactate	310 mg	K^+	4 mEq	Lactate$^-$	28 mEq
Na($C_3H_5O_3$)					
KCl	30 mg	Ca^{++}	3 mEq		
$CaCl_2$	20 mg				
	Totals:		137 mEq		137 mEq

Exact calculation cannot be done because the GAWs in Table 6.1 are only approximate. Therefore, the answers will only approximate the 137 mEq total cations and 137 total anions on the label.

Step 1   Make a chart so that the final numbers of cations and anions can be added. There are several compounds containing sodium and chloride, all of which must be added to get the total number of each of the ions in the Ringer's lactate. The chart can by filled in as the figuring is done.

Proof of Ringer's Lactate Label

	mEq Cations			mEq Anions	
	Na^+	K^+	Ca^{++}	Cl^-	$(C_3H_5O_3)^-$
NaCl					
Na($C_3H_5O_3$)					
KCl					
$CaCl_2$					
Total:					

Step 2   The first electrolyte on the label is NaCl, of which there are 600 mg in each 100 ml of solution.

$$\text{total mg of NaCl in 1,000 ml} = \frac{600 \text{ mg} \times 10 = 6,000 \text{ mg}}{100 \text{ ml} \times 10 = 1,000 \text{ ml}}$$

$$\text{total mEq of NaCl in 1,000 ml} = \frac{\text{total mg NaCl/1,000 ml}}{\text{mEq weight of NaCl}}$$

$$\text{mEq weight of NaCl} = (23 \text{ mg} + 35 \text{ mg})/(1 \times 1) = 58 \text{ mg/mEq}$$

$$\text{number of mEq of NaCl/1,000 ml} = 6,000 \text{ mg} \div 58 \text{ mg/mEq}$$

$$= \overset{103}{\cancel{6,000} \text{ mg}} \times \frac{\text{mEq}}{\cancel{58} \text{ mg}}$$

$$= 103 \text{ mEq NaCl}$$

Therefore:

103 mEq Na$^+$ + 103 mEq Cl$^-$ = 103 mEq NaCl in 1,000 ml of Ringer's lactate

The chart for NaCl can be completed. (An example is at the end of the chapter.)

Step 3 The next electrolyte in the label is Na($C_3H_5O_3$). The label indicates that there are 310 mg of Na lactate in each 100 ml of the solution.

$$\text{total mg of Na lactate in the 1,000 ml} = \frac{310 \text{ mg} \times 10}{100 \text{ ml} \times 10} = \frac{3,100 \text{ mg}}{1,000 \text{ ml}}$$

$$\text{mEq weight of Na lactate} = (23 + 36 + 5 + 48 \text{ mg})/(1 \times 1)$$

$$= 112 \text{ mg}/(1 \times 1) = 112 \text{ mg/mEq}$$

$$\text{number of mEq of Na}(C_3H_5O_3)/1,000 \text{ ml} = 3,100 \text{ mg} \div 112 \text{ mg/mEq}$$

$$= \overset{28}{\cancel{3,100 \text{ mg}}} \times \frac{\text{mEq}}{\cancel{112 \text{ mg}}}$$

$$= 28 \text{ mEq Na lactate in 1,000 ml}$$

Therefore:

28 mEq Na$^+$ + 28 mEq $(C_3H_5O_3)^-$ = 28 mEq Na($C_3H_5O_3$)

The chart for Na$^+$ and $(C_3H_5O_3)^-$ can be completed.

Step 4 The next electrolyte on the label is KCl, of which there are 30 mg in each 100 ml of solution.

$$\text{total mg of KCl in 1,000 ml} = \frac{30 \text{ mg} \times 10}{100 \text{ ml} \times 10} = \frac{300 \text{ mg}}{1,000 \text{ ml}}$$

$$\text{mEq weight of KCl} = (39 + 35 \text{ mg})/(1 \times 1) = 74 \text{ mg/mEq}$$

$$\text{number of mEq of KCl}/1,000 \text{ ml of Ringer's lactate} = 300 \text{ mg} \div 74 \text{ mg/mEq}$$

$$= \overset{4}{\cancel{300 \text{ mg}}} \times \frac{\text{mEq}}{\cancel{74 \text{ mg}}} = 4 \text{ mEq KCl}/1,000 \text{ ml}$$

Therefore:

4 mEq K$^+$ + 4 mEq Cl$^-$ = 4 mEq KCl

The chart for KCl can be completed.

Step 5 The last electrolyte listed on the label is 20 mg of $CaCl_2$ in 100 ml.

$$\frac{20 \text{ mg} \times 10}{100 \text{ ml} \times 10} = \frac{200 \text{ mg}}{1,000 \text{ ml}}$$

$$\text{mEq weight of CaCl}_2 = (40 + 35 + 35) \text{ mg}/2 = 110 \text{ mg}/2 = 55 \text{ mg/mEq}$$

number of mEq of $CaCl_2$ in 1,000 ml of Ringer's lactate

$$= 200 \text{ mg} \div 55 \text{ mg/mEq} = \cancel{200 \text{ mg}} \times \frac{\overset{3.6}{mEq}}{\cancel{55 \text{ mg}}} = 3.6 \text{ mEq of } CaCl_2$$

The chart for $CaCl_2$ can be completed.

Step 6   Add the totals in the chart. Compare them with the label on the Ringer's lactate bottle. The results are quite close.

Proof of Ringer's Lactate Label

	mEq Cations			mEq Anions	
	Na^+	K^+	Ca^{++}	Cl^-	$(C_3H_5O_3)^-$
NaCl	103			103	
$Na(C_3H_5O_3)$	28				28
KCl		4		4	
$CaCl_2$			3.6	3.6	
Total	131 +	4 +	3.6	110.6 +	28

138.6 mEq cations = 138.6 mEq anions

Chapter 10
OSMOSIS,
OSMOTIC PRESSURE
OF SOLUTIONS,
OSMOLS,
OSMOLALITY

OSMOSIS

A membrane separating two fluid compartments that is permeable to water molecules, but not to some of the dissolved solutes, is known as a semipermeable membrane. If the concentration of nondiffusible solutes is greater on one side of the membrane than it is on the other side, water molecules will pass through the semipermeable membrane toward the side with the greater concentration of nondiffusible solute. This process is known as osmosis.

Figure 10.1, diagram 1, represents a U-tube with a porous membrane at the bottom separating compartments A and B. The B side of the U-tube is filled with pure water, and the A side is filled with a solution of 5% dextrose in water (5% D/W). Both sides contain the same volume of fluid. The membrane is impermeable to dextrose, but water can flow freely through its pores. After a time, the U-tube will look like diagram 2. Water has flowed from the B side to the A side, where it has greatly diluted the dextrose solution.

Why Osmosis Occurs

Since the temperature is the same on both sides of the semipermeable membrane, the chemical activity or motion of all the molecules is the same on both sides. If the membrane had holes large enough so that the dextrose molecules could go through them, after a time the number of dextrose and water molecules would be the same on both sides of the membrane, i.e., the dextrose concentration would be the same in B as it is in A. (This process is known as diffusion.)

However, the holes in the membrane in Fig. 10.1 are too small

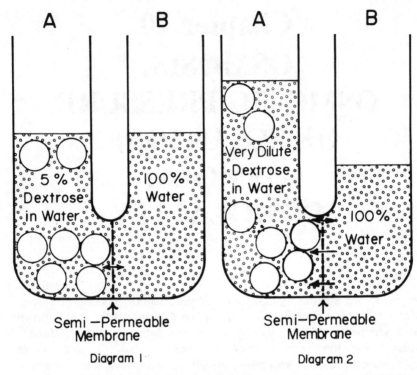

Figure 10.1. Osmosis. Compartment A of Diagram 1 contains a solution of 5% D/W. Compartment B contains pure water molecules (small circles). The dextrose molecules in A (large circles) are too large to pass through the pores of the semi-permeable membrane that separates the 2 compartments. Diagram 2 represents the appearance of the U-tube after a time interval.

for the dextrose molecules to flow through them. Under these circumstances, the holes on the B side are bombarded only by water molecules, but the holes on the A side are bombarded by both dextrose and water molecules. More water molecules strike the holes on the B side than on the A side, so more water goes through the membrane from B to A than in the opposite direction. This net rate of diffusion of water molecules from the water side to the solute side is known as the rate of osmosis.

Figure 10.1, diagram 2, shows that the volume of water in the A compartment has increased as much as it has decreased on the B side. The process of water going from B into A will continue until a point of equilibrium is reached. This point of equilibrium is reached when the weight of the water and solute on the A side of the membrane becomes just enough greater than the weight of the water on the B side to prevent any more water from crossing the membrane from B into A. Thus, the mechanical or hydrostatic pressure of the solute and water on the A side of the membrane opposes the flow of water across the membrane from the B side. This pressure is known as the osmotic pressure of the 5% D/W. Thus, the point of equilibrium is reached when the hydrostatic pressure is the same as the osmotic pressure. The water stops flowing from B to A at that point.

OSMOTIC PRESSURE OF SOLUTIONS

Figure 10.2 illustrates osmotic pressure. Osmosis of water molecules from compartment B into compartment A through a membrane that is impermeable to dextrose can be prevented by applying a mechanical force by the plunger on top of the solution in compartment A. The exact amount of pressure required by the plunger to stop the water from flowing from B into A measures the osmotic pressure of the solution.

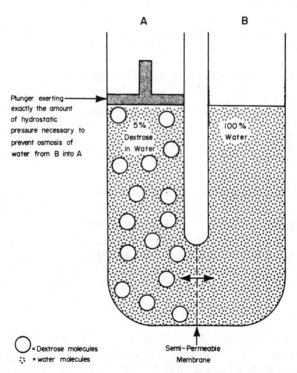

Figure 10.2. Osmotic Pressure. The exact amount of mechanical or hydrostatic pressure required by the plunger to stop the water from flowing from B into A through a membrane that is impermeable to dextrose molecules is known as the osmotic pressure of that solution.

Technical Definition of Osmotic Pressure

That pressure in millimeters of mercury which, when applied to a solution, will *just* prevent the entrance of the solvent into it through a semipermeable membrane is the osmotic pressure of that solution. (Millimeters of mercury, abbreviated mmHg, is a unit of weight used in physics and chemistry to measure pressure.)

The amount of osmotic pressure that a solution exerts depends upon the concentration of the solute. For example: 1% D/W has less osmotic pressure than a solution of 2% D/W; 2% D/W has less osmotic pressure than a solution of 5% D/W; and 5% D/W exerts half the amount of osmotic pressure as that exerted by 10% D/W.

Figure 10.2 shows that a 5% D/W solution requires a certain amount of mechanical or hydrostatic pressure by the plunger to prevent osmosis of water from side B into side A. If there were only 1% D/W in the A side, just one-fifth as much pressure by the plunger would be required to prevent osmosis of water from compartment B into compartment A. Conversely, if there were 10% D/W in the A compartment, twice as much pressure by the plunger would be required to prevent osmosis of water from compartment B into compartment A.

Relationship of GMW to Percentage of Solution

If the beakers in Figure 10.3 are compared, the relationship between the GMW of a solute and its percentage in a solution can be seen. Beakers A and B represent solutions that are identical in weights of solute because both of them are 5% solutions. One liter of a 5% solution of any solute (drug, chemical, etc.) contains 50 g of that solute. (See Chap. 2.)

However, the number of molecules in a liter of 5% D/W is not the same as in a liter of 5% alcohol. This fact is proved by the GMW of each substance. A GMW of dextrose weighs 180 g, and a GMW of alcohol weighs 46 g. A GMW of any compound contains the same number of molecules as a GMW of any other compound. The number of molecules in a GMW of any substance is 6.02×10^{23}. (Review Chap. 6, which discusses Avogadro's law and number.) The number of molecules in these two substances can be determined by taking the following steps:

Step 1   In beaker A of Figure 10.3, there are 50 g of dextrose in 1 L of water; 1 GMW of dextrose weighs 180 g. What part of 1 GMW of dextrose is there in 1 L of 5% D/W?

$$50 \text{ g} \div 180 \text{ g/GMW} = \overset{.28}{\cancel{50} \text{ g}} \times \frac{\text{GMW}}{\cancel{180} \text{ g}} = .28 \text{ GMW of dextrose}$$

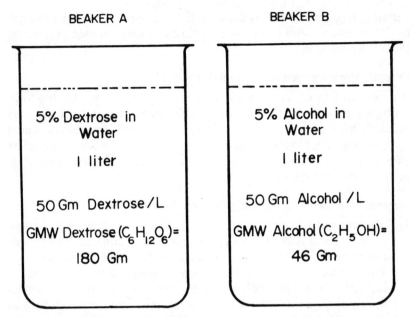

BEAKER A

BEAKER B

5% Dextrose in Water

I liter

50 Gm Dextrose/L

GMW Dextrose $(C_6H_{12}O_6)=$ 180 Gm

5% Alcohol in Water

I liter

50 Gm Alcohol /L

GMW Alcohol $(C_2H_5OH)=$ 46 Gm

Figure 10.3. GMW and Percentages of Solutions. Beakers comparing the GMWs of dextrose and alcohol in relation to identical 5% concentrations (See text)

Step 2   How many molecules are there in .28 GMW of dextrose?

$$\frac{6.02 \times 10^{23} \text{ molecules}}{GMW} \times .28 \ GMW = 1.69 \times 10^{23} \text{ molecules of dextrose}$$

Step 3   In beaker B of Figure 10.3, there are 50 g of alcohol in 1 L of water; 1 GMW of alcohol weighs 46 g. How many GMW of alcohol are there in 1 L of 5% alcohol in water?

$$50 \text{ g} \div 46 \text{ g/GMW} = 50 \text{g} \times \frac{GMW}{46 \text{ g}} = 1.1 \text{ GMW of alcohol}$$

Step 4   How many molecules are there in 1.1 GMW of alcohol?

$$\frac{6.02 \times 10^{23} \text{ molecules}}{GMW} \times 1.1 \ GMW = 6.622 \times 10^{23} \text{ molecules of alcohol}$$

Step 5   Compare the osmotic pressure of the two solutions.

$$\frac{6.622 \times 10^{23} \text{ molecules in 1 L of 5% alcohol}}{1.69 \times 10^{23} \text{ molecules in 1 L of 5% dextrose}}$$

= 3.92 times as many molecules in the beaker of

5% alcohol as in the beaker of 5% dextrose

Since osmotic pressure is caused by the number of molecules in a solution, it is obvious in this situation that the osmotic pressure exerted by 1 L of 5% alcohol is almost four times as great as that exerted by the 5% dextrose solution.

Osmotic Pressure Exerted by Ionizing Solutions

If an electrolyte ionizes in a solution, and if the ions are too big to go through the pores of the semipermeable membrane, i.e., if they are nondiffusible, each ion individually exerts osmotic pressure, because each ion can effectively "plug" one pore in the membrane. Each ion exerts as much osmotic pressure as one molecule of any nonionizing, nondiffusible substance.

General Statements Concerning Osmotic Pressure

1. The amount of osmotic pressure that one molecule of a nonionizing, nondiffusible substance exerts is the same as that of one molecule of any other non-ionizing, nondiffusible substance.
2. The difference between molecules of nonionizing substances is primarily in weight, rather than in size. One nonionizing protein molecule with a GMW of 70,000 g has the same osmotic effect as one molecule of dextrose with a GMW of 180 g. Each molecule of dextrose plugs a pore in the semipermeable membrane as effectively as does one molecule of protein. Compare the weight of a marble with that of a ping-pong ball of the same size. Either one of them can effectively plug a hole of the same diameter.
3. The amount of osmotic pressure that one ion of a nondiffusible electrolyte exerts is the same as that of one molecule of any nonionizing, nondiffusible substance, or the same as that of one ion of any other ionizing, nondiffusible substance.
4. One molecule of a nondiffusible, nonionizing substance or one ion of a nondiffusible electrolyte, is known as one solute particle that exerts osmotic pressure.

OSMOLS

A method is needed for measuring osmotic pressure. The unit of measure for osmotic activity is known as the osmol. Since it is the number of particles that creates the osmotic pressure of a solution, the osmol adds, or counts, the number of solute particles in the solution. The concentration of osmotically active particles in a solution is generally designated as the number of osmols per liter of solution. The osmotic pressure of a solution can easily be calculated if the number of osmols per liter is known.

An osmol is directly related to the GMW of a substance, and

equals 6.02×10^{23} particles of dissolved solute that cannot diffuse through a semipermeable membrane. These particles of solute may be a combination of several different kinds of nondiffusible ions and molecules in a solution.

Definition of an Osmol

One GMW of a dissolved, nonionizing, nondiffusible solute equals one osmol (Osm). One GMW of such a solute contains 6.02×10^{23} molecules.

One GAW of an electrolyte that ionizes in solution equals 1 Osm. One GAW of such a solute contains 6.02×10^{23} ions.

Examples

When osmotic pressure is being calculated, all the nondiffusible molecules, and all the nondiffusible ions in a solution must be added. Each particle exerts the same amount of osmotic pressure. Therefore: 1 Na^+ ion has the same osmotic effect as one nonionizing molecule of dextrose; 1 Ca^{++} ion has the same osmotic effect as 1 Na^+ ion, or one dextrose molecule; 1 $CaCl_2$ molecule ionizes into three ions—1 Ca^{++} and 2 Cl^-—exerting three times as much osmotic pressure as does one molecule of dextrose, simply because $CaCl_2$ ionizes when placed in water and exerts three particles of osmotic pressure; 1 NaCl molecule exerts two particles of osmotic pressure; 1 Na^+ ion exerts one particle of osmotic pressure; and one glucose molecule exerts one particle of osmotic pressure.

Summary

The unit of measure for osmotic activity is the osmol (Osm). The osmol expresses the number of solute particles in a solution, because it is the number of solute particles that creates its osmotic pressure.

When speaking of the osmotic pressure of a solution, the concentration of osmotically active particles is generally given in osmols per liter of solution.

One GMW of a dissolved, nondiffusible, and nonionizing substance equals 1 Osm.

If a substance ionizes into two particles, and the particles are nondiffusible, 1 GMW of that substance equals 2 Osm. An example is:

$$NaCl \rightarrow Na^+ + Cl^-$$

When the substance ionizes, each molecule splits into two particles. Therefore, it exerts twice as much osmotic pressure as one molecule of a non-ionizing substance.

$$1 \text{ GAW Na}^+ = 1 \text{ Osm}$$
$$1 \text{ GAW Cl}^- = 1 \text{ Osm}$$
$$1 \text{ GMW NaCl} = 2 \text{ Osm}$$
$$.5 \text{ GMW NaCl} = 1 \text{ Osm}$$

Each solute particle in a solution decreases the molecular concentration of the water by exactly the same amount regardless of the weight of the particle. For this reason, expressing the concentration of the solute in a solution in terms of gram weight, i.e., g% or g/L is of absolutely no value when calculating osmotic pressure of a solution.

MEASURING THE OSMOTIC PRESSURE OR OSMOLALITY OF SOLUTIONS

Definition of Osmolality

The osmolality of a solution is the number of osmols, or the fraction of 1 Osm that is dissolved in a given unit of solvent, usually 1 L. The osmolality of a solution is generally expressed as osmols per liter of solvent.

The osmotic pressure of a solution is that pressure in mmHg which, when applied to a solution, will just prevent the entrance of the solvent into it through a semipermeable membrane. To expand this definition it can be stated that 1 GMW of any nonionizing, nondiffusible solute, dissolved in 22.4 L of water at 0° centigrade (C), has an osmotic pressure of 760 mmHg, and contains 6.02×10^{23} particles.

The *osmolality* of the nonionizing solution described above is 1 GMW or one osmol per 22.4 liters of water (generally expressed, 1 Osm/22.4 L). It has an osmotic pressure of 760 mmHg, which is commonly known as 1 atmosphere (atm) of pressure.

Example 1

In Figure 10.4, diagram 1, 180 g (or 1 GMW) of dextrose is dissolved in 22.4 L of water, and poured into compartment A of a U-tube. It is separated from 22.4 L of pure water in side B of the U-tube by a membrane that is impermeable to dextrose molecules. In addition, 1 atm of pressure (760 mmHg) is exerted by the plunger on top of the solution in compartment A. This is exactly the amount of mechanical, or hydrostatic, pressure needed to prevent the osmosis of water from B into A through the semipermeable membrane. (If more than 760 mmHg pressure were exerted by the plunger, the water would flow from compartment A into compartment B until an equilibrium was reached with the additional pressure.)

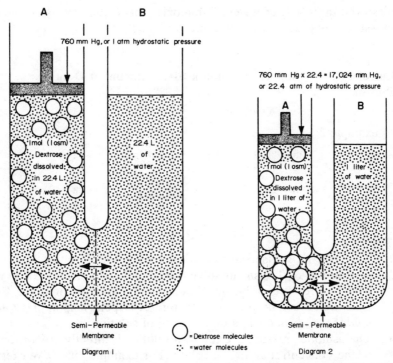

Figure 10.4. Osmotic pressure exerted by 1 GMW of dextrose dissolved in 22.4 L of water (Diagram 1), and by 1 GMW of dextrose dissolved in 1 L of water (Diagram 2), when compartments A and B are separated by a membrane that is impermeable to dextrose molecules

Avogadro's law states that this 1 GMW of dextrose contains 6.02×10^{23} molecules or particles, and that this number of particles equals 1 Osm. If this 1 Osm, or 6.02×10^{23} particles, is dissolved in exactly 22.4 L of water, the solution will exert an osmotic pressure of exactly 1 atm (760 mmHg).

Example 2

If 1 GMW of dextrose (1 Osm) is dissolved in 1 L of water, the solution will exert an osmotic pressure of 760 mmHg × 22.4, or 17,024 mmHg at 0°C, because it has been concentrated 22.4 times. In Figure 10.4, diagram 2, 180 g (or 1 GMW or 1 Osm) of dextrose is dissolved in only 1 L of water. It is separated from 1 L of pure water in compartment B of the U-tube by a membrane that is impermeable to dextrose molecules. This situation requires that 22.4 times as much pressure be exerted by the plunger to prevent osmosis of water from B into A, as was required when the same amount of solute was dissolved in 22.4 L of water. Commonly, this 17,024 mmHg osmotic pressure is expressed as 22.4 atm of pressure.

Calculating the Number of atm in a Given Amount of Osmotic Pressure

$$atm = mmHg \div 760 \ mmHg/atm$$

In example 2:

$$atm = 17,024 \ mmHg \div 760 \ mmHg/atm$$

$$atm = \overset{22.4}{\cancel{17,024}} \ \cancel{mmHg} \times \frac{atm}{\cancel{760 \ mmHg}} = 22.4 \ atm$$

Summary

1. The term 1 Osm is used to express 6.02×10^{23} particles.
2. A solution of 1 Osm dissolved in 22.4 L of solvent exerts an osmotic pressure of 760 mmHg or 1 atm of osmotic pressure.
3. Osmotic force, or pressure, therefore, depends upon the *total number of particles* in a unit volume of solution.
4. The osmotic pressure exerted by a solution is directly proportional to the concentration of the solute. For example, 5% D/W exerts five times as much osmotic pressure as does 1% D/W.
5. For a given amount of solute, the osmotic pressure is inversely proportional to the volume of solvent. For example, if 1 g of any non-ionizing solute, dissolved in 1 L of water, exerts one arbitrary unit of osmotic pressure, it can be calculated that:

$$1 \ g/L = 1 \ unit \ of \ pressure$$

$$50 \ g/L = 50 \ units \ of \ pressure$$

$$50 \ g/2 \ L = 25 \ g/L = 25 \ units \ of \ pressure$$

$$50 \ g/.5 \ L = 100 \ g/L = 100 \ units \ of \ pressure$$

Here it is demonstrated that the less the volume of solvent used to dissolve a given amount of solute, the more the osmotic pressure that will be exerted by the solution, and conversely, the more the volume of solvent used to dissolve a given amount of solute, the less the osmotic pressure that will be exerted by that solution.

6. The fact that 1 Osm of a given nondiffusible solute, dissolved in 22.4 L of water, creates an osmotic pressure of 760 mmHg, serves only as a point of reference for comparison with other concentrations of the same solute.

Osmolality of Ionized, Nondiffusible Solutions

Example 1

In Figure 10.5, diagram 1, 58 g (or 1 GMW) of NaCl is dissolved in 22.4 L of water, and poured into compartment A of a U-tube. It is separated from 22.4 L of water in the B side of the U-tube by a semipermeable membrane that is impermeable to NaCl ions. In addition, 2 atm of pressure, or 1520 mmHg pressure (760 mmHg × 2) is exerted by the plunger on top of the solution in compartment A. This is exactly the amount of mechanical or hydrostatic pressure needed to prevent osmosis of water from compartment B into compartment A through the semipermeable membrane. One GMW NaCl contains 6.02 × 10²³ molecules. Each molecule ionizes into two ions, or particles. The number of particles has doubled. Therefore, 1 GMW of NaCl equals 2 Osm; 6.02 × 10²³ molecules ionize into 2(6.02) × 10²³ or 12.04 × 10²³ ions.

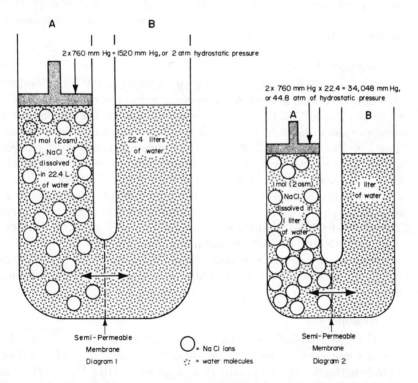

Figure 10.5. Osmotic pressure exerted by 1 GMW or 2 osmols of NaCl dissolved in 22.4 L of water (Diagram 1), and by 1 GMW or 2 osmols of NaCl dissolved in 1 L of water (Diagram 2), when compartments A and B are separated by a membrane that is impermeable to NaCl ions

The actual osmotic pressure exerted by these 12.04×10^{23} particles (or 2 Osm) depends upon the volume of solvent in which the particles are dissolved.

Example 2

If 1 GMW of NaCl (2 Osm) is dissolved in 1 L of water, the solution will exert an osmotic pressure of 760 mmHg $\times$ 22.4 $\times$ 2 (34,048 mmHg) at 0°C. In Figure 10.5, diagram 2, 58 g (or 1 GMW) of NaCl is dissolved in only 1 L of water, and poured into compartment A of a U-tube. It is separated from 1 L of water in the B side of the U-tube by a semipermeable membrane that is impermeable to NaCl ions. The solution has been concentrated 22.4 times. This situation requires that 22.4 times as much pressure be exerted by the plunger on top of the solution in the A compartment, to prevent osmosis of water from B into A, as was required when the same amount of solute was dissolved in 22.4 L of water. Commonly, this 34,048 mmHg osmotic pressure is expressed as 44.8 atm of pressure. Thus, 12.04×10^{23} particles (2 Osm) dissolved in 1 L of water, exert 44.8 atm or 34,048 mmHg osmotic pressure at 0°C.

Example 3

In Figure 10.6, diagram 1, 110 g (or 1 GMW) of $CaCl_2$ is dissolved in 22.4 L of water, and poured into compartment A of a U-tube. It is separated from 22.4 L of water in the B side of the U-tube by a semipermeable membrane that is impermeable to $CaCl_2$ ions. It will take 3 $\times$ 760 mmHg or 2,280 mmHg (3 atm) pressure by the plunger on top of solution A to prevent the osmosis of water from compartment B into compartment A, through a semipermeable membrane. In 1 GMW $CaCl_2$ there are 6.02×10^{23} molecules. Each molecule ionizes into three particles, or ions. The number of particles has tripled. Therefore, 1 GMW of $CaCl_2$ = 3 Osm; 6.02×10^{23} molecules ionizes into $3(6.02) \times 10^{23}$ or 18.06×10^{23} ions.

The actual osmotic pressure exerted by these 18.06×10^{23} particles (3 Osm) depends upon the volume of water in which the particles are dissolved.

Example 4

If 1 GMW of $CaCl_2$ (3 Osm) is dissolved in only 1 L of water, the solution will exert an osmotic pressure of 760 mmHg $\times$ 22.4 $\times$ 3 or 51,072 mmHg at 0°C. In Figure 10.6, diagram 2, 110 g (or 1 GMW) of $CaCl_2$ is dissolved in only 1 L of water, and poured into compartment A of a U-tube. It is separated from 1 L of water in the B side of the U-tube by a semipermeable membrane that is impermeable to $CaCl_2$

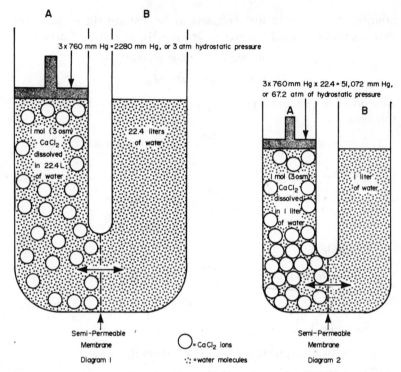

Figure 10.6.   Osmotic pressure exerted by 1 GMW or 3 osmols of CaCl$_2$ dissolved in 22.4 L of water (Diagram 1), and by 1 GMW or 3 osmols of CaCl$_2$ dissolved in 1 L of water (Diagram 2), when compartments A and B are separated by a membrane that is impermeable to CaCl$_2$ ions

ions. The solution has been concentrated 22.4 times. This situation requires that 22.4 times as much pressure be exerted by the plunger on top of the solution in compartment A, to prevent osmosis of water from B into A, as was required when the same amount of solute was dissolved in 22.4 L of water. Commonly, this 51,072 mmHg pressure is expressed as 67.2 atm of pressure. Thus, 18.06×10^{23} particles (3 Osm), dissolved in 1 L of solvent, exert 67.2 atm, or 51,072 mmHg osmotic pressure at 0°C.

Summary

For any nondiffusible solute, 1 Osm exerts an osmotic pressure of 1 atm *only if* it is dissolved in 22.4 L of water. The mathematics may be made simpler by this statement, but it is the most confusing factor of the entire concept. There is no magic in the 22.4 L, or in the fact that atmospheric pressure just happens to be 760 mmHg at sea level, or that scientists elected to refer to 760 mmHg as 1 atm of pressure.

$$760 \text{ mmHg} = 1 \text{ atm pressure}$$

$$1 \text{ Osm}/22.4 \text{ L} = 1 \text{ atm of pressure}$$

Any problem concerning osmotic pressure can be calculated from just this data:

$$\text{osmotic pressure of } \frac{1 \text{ Osm}}{22.4 \text{ L}} = 760 \text{ mmHg or 1 atm at } 0°C$$

Example 1

$$\text{osmotic pressure of } \frac{2 \text{ Osm}}{22.4 \text{ L}} = 760 \text{ mmHg} \times 2$$

$$= 1{,}520 \text{ mmHg or 2 atm}$$

Example 2

$$\text{osmotic pressure of } \frac{1 \text{ Osm}}{L} = 760 \text{ mmHg} \times 22.4$$

$$= 17{,}024 \text{ mmHg or 22.4 atm}$$

Example 3

$$\text{osmotic pressure of } \frac{1 \text{ Osm}}{2 \text{ L}} = 760 \text{ mmHg} \times \frac{22.4}{2}$$

$$= 8{,}512 \text{ mmHg or 11.2 atm}$$

Example 4

$$\text{osmotic pressure of } \frac{1 \text{ Osm}}{.5 \text{ L}} = 760 \text{ mmHg} \times \frac{22.4}{.5}$$

$$= 34{,}048 \text{ mmHg or 44.8 atm}$$

Example 5

$$\text{osmotic pressure of } \frac{.5 \text{ Osm}}{22.4 \text{ L}} = 760 \text{ mmHg} \times .5$$

$$= 380.0 \text{ mmHg or .5 atm}$$

Example 6

$$\text{osmotic pressure of } \frac{3 \text{ Osm}}{L} = 760 \text{ mmHg} \times 3 \times 22.4$$

$$= 51{,}072 \text{ mmHg or 67.2 atm}$$

Table 10.1 is a chart summarizing the above relationships. It shows that:

1. For the same gram weight of a given solute, the more volume, the less osmotic pressure; the less volume, the more osmotic pressure.

Table 10.1 Osmotic Pressure of Various Solutions

Basic Equation: Osmotic pressure of 1 Osm/22.4 L = 760 mmHg ≡ 1 atm

If 1 GMW of a non-ionizing solute (which is 1 Osm, or 6.02 × 10²³ particles) is dissolved in:

.5 L of water,

$$\frac{1\,Osm}{.5\,L} = 760\,mmHg \times \frac{22.4}{.5} = 34{,}048\,mmHg \equiv 44.8\,atm$$

Osmotic pressure of 1 Osm/.5 L = 34,048 mmHg ≡ 44.8 atm

1.0 L of water,

$$\frac{1\,Osm}{1.0\,L} = 760\,mmHg \times \frac{22.4}{1.0} = 17{,}024\,mmHg = 22.4\,atm$$

Osmotic pressure of 1 Osm/L = 17,024 mmHg ≡ 22.4 atm

2.0 L of water,

$$\frac{1\,Osm}{2.0\,L} = 760\,mmHg \times \frac{\overset{11.2}{22.4}}{2.0} = 8512\,mmHg \equiv 11.2\,atm$$

Osmotic pressure of 1 Osm/2 L = 8512 mmHg ≡ 11.2 atm

or

If .5 GMW of a monovalent ionizing solute (which is 1 Osm, or 6.02 × 10²³ particles) is dissolved in:

22.4 L of water,

$$\frac{1\,Osm}{22.4\,L} = 760\,mmHg \times \frac{22.4}{22.4} = 760\,mmHg = 1\,atm$$

Osmotic pressure of 1 Osm/22.4 L = 760 mmHg ≡ 1 atm

or

If .33 GMW of a bivalent ionizing solute (which is 1 Osm, or 6.02 × 10²³ particles) is dissolved in:

2240 L of water,

$$\frac{1\,Osm}{2{,}240\,L} = 760\,mmHg \times \frac{\overset{.01}{22.4}}{2{,}240} = 7.6\,mmHg = .01\,atm$$

Osmotic pressure of 1 Osm/2,240 L = 7.6 mmHg ≡ .01 atm

2.   1 Osm/22.4 L = an osmotic pressure of 760 mmHg, or 1 atm
     This equation serves only as a point of reference for comparison
     with other concentrations of the same amount of solute.
3.   1 Osm =
     a.   1 GMW of a nonionizing substance
     b.   .5 GMW of an ionizing monovalent substance, such as NaCl,
          because, when placed in water, each molecule splits into two
          ions or particles
     c.   .33 GMW of an ionizing bivalent substance, such as $CaCl_2$,
          because, when placed in water, each molecule splits into three
          ions or particles

Osmolality of Body Fluids at Body Temperature

When 1 GMW of any nonionizing substance is dissolved in 22.4 L of
water at 0°C it has an osmotic pressure of 760 mmHg.

Absolute 0 is the temperature at which all atomic and molecular
motion stops. It is −273°C; 0°C is 273°C warmer than absolute 0.

Since human beings have a normal body temperature of 98.6°F,
or 37°C, these figures must be adjusted to reflect this warm temperature.

A scientist named Gay-Lussac is credited with the following law:
If the volume of a gas remains constant, the pressure varies directly
with the absolute temperature 1/273 for each degree centigrade. Solutes in solutions abide by this law. At 0°C (273°C warmer than absolute
zero), the osmotic pressure exerted by 1 Osm of solute/L of water is
273/273 × 760 mmHg × 22.4 = 17,024 mmHg.

At 37°C (normal body temperature), the osmotic pressure of 1
Osm of solute/L of solvent is [(273 + 37)/273] × 760 mmHg × 22.4 =
19,331 mmHg.

These figures must be reduced to a useful size. *Milliosmols*
(mOsm) are used when referring to small osmotic pressures within the
human body. Just as:

$$1,000 \text{ mg} = 1 \text{ g}$$

$$1,000 \text{ mOsm} = 1 \text{ Osm}$$

$$.001 \text{ Osm} = 1 \text{ mOsm}$$

Since, at 37°C:

$$\text{osmotic pressure of 1 Osm of solute/L} = 19,331 \text{ mmHg,}$$

$$\text{osmotic pressure of 1,000 mOsm of solute/L} = 19,331 \text{ mmHg}$$

$$\text{osmotic pressure of 1 mOsm/L} = 19.3 \text{ mmHg}$$

Body Fluid Osmotic Pressures

Biological scientists measured the osmotic concentration of normal body fluids and found them to be about 300 mOsm/L (.3 Osm/L). Since 1 mOsm/L of water creates an osmotic pressure of 19.3 mmHg at 37°C:

$$\text{osmotic pressure of 300 mOsm/L} = 19.3 \text{ mmHg} \times 300 = 5790 \text{ mmHg}$$

There are three major compartmentalized fluids in the body, separated by semipermeable membranes. They are plasma of the blood; intracellular fluid (ICF), which is the fluid that is found within each one of the many different kinds of cells that make up the body; and interstitial fluid (ISF), which is the fluid between all the cells. The plasma and the interstitial fluids make up the extracellular fluid (ECF).

Figure 10.7 represents the three major fluid compartments in the body, and the respective osmotic pressures that exist within each compartment. The vast amount of osmotic pressure shown in each of the three compartments illustrates the huge force that the "plunger" (hydrostatic pressure) would have to exert to prevent osmosis, if pure water were on one side of a membrane that separates the compartments. Figure 10.7 shows, however, that the pressures in the three compartments are identical (or are in equilibrium), except for an extra 25 mmHg that exists in the plasma. This 25 mmHg osmotic pressure is caused by the plasma proteins, which exist only in the blood. The

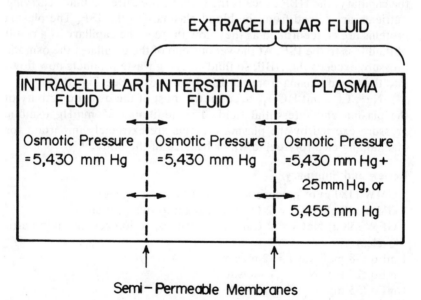

Figure 10.7.   Osmotic Pressure Within Various Body Fluid Compartments (See text)

capillary membrane is impermeable to the plasma proteins, and, therefore, the plasma proteins are very important for controlling fluid exchanges between the blood and interstitial fluid.

Since the plasma proteins normally have an osmotic concentration of 1.3 mOsm/L of plasma, it can be calculated that

osmotic pressure of 1.3 mOsm/L = 19.3 mmHg × 1.3 = 25 mmHg

Therefore, the osmotic pressure of these plasma proteins is about 25 mmHg.

(The student may notice the discrepancy between the 5790 mmHg osmotic pressure calculated above for body fluids, and the 5430 mmHg osmotic pressure shown in Figure 10.7. The round figure, 300 mOsm/L osmotic concentration, was used in the original explanation. In reality, the osmotic concentration of body fluids is closer to 280–283 mOsm/L, but varies from tissue to tissue.)

Fluid Dynamics at the Capillary

The hydrostatic blood pressure (HBP) is a mechanical force originating with each heart beat. It is analogous to the plunger in the U-tube diagrams. The HBP pushes fluids out of the blood plasma into the ISF at the arterial end of the capillary. The osmotic pressure exerted by the plasma proteins causes osmosis of fluids into the blood plasma from the ISF at the venous end of the capillary. At the arterial end of the capillary, the HBP exceeds the osmotic pressure, so fluids carrying nutrients are forced from the blood plasma into the ISF. The plasma proteins are concentrated as they flow through the capillary as a result of fluid loss to the ISF. At the venous end of the capillary, the osmotic pressure exceeds the HBP, so fluid carrying waste products now flows into the blood plasma from the ISF by osmosis. See Fig. 10.8.

Na^+, Cl^-, and HCO_3^- account for most of the osmotic activity of the plasma and interstitial fluid. The additional 25 mmHg osmotic pressure exerted by the plasma proteins are extremely important for maintaining electrolyte and water balance of the body.

Review and Summary

1 GMW (180 g) of glucose = 1 Osm (does not ionize)
1 GMW (58 g) NaCl = 2 Osm (ionizes into two particles)
1 GEW (58 g) NaCl = 2 Osm (monovalent, so ionizes into two particles)
1 mEq (58 mg) NaCl = 2 mOsm
1 mEq (23 mg) Na^+ = 1 mOsm
1 mEq (35 mg) Cl^- = 1 mOsm
.5 mEq Na^+ = .5 mOsm

Interstitial Fluid

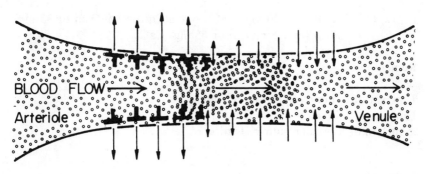

Interstitial Fluid

Figure 10.8. Diagram of Fluid Exchange at the Capillary

Code

— — — Semi-permeable membrane, impermeable to plasma proteins

"Plungers" Hydrostatic blood pressure exerted on the inside of the entire length of all blood vessels. It varies, becoming progressively less as blood flows from the arteriole through the capillary to the venule.

Plasma proteins, which are too large to go through the pores of the capillary membrane. They become more concentrated as fluid is forced out of the capillary into the interstitial fluid by the hydrostatic blood pressure. The plasma proteins are diluted as fluid comes into the blood at the venous end of the capillary by osmosis. Fluids diffuse in an attempt to reach equilibrium, but since the blood is in constant motion, equilibrium is never reached.

←——→ Arrows indicate the direction of fluid flow.

.5 mEq Cl^- = .5 mOsm
.5 mEq NaCl = 1 mOsm

Therefore:

1 mEq (or 1 mOsm or 23 mg) Na^+ + 1 mEq (or 1 mOsm or 35 mg) Cl^-
 → 1 mEq (or 2 mOsm or 58 mg) NaCl
1 GMW (110 g) $CaCl_2$ = 3 Osm (each molecule ionizes into three particles)
1 GEW (55 g) $CaCl_2$ = 1.5 Osm
1 mEq (55 mg) $CaCl_2$ = 1.5 mOsm
1 GAW (40 g) Ca^{++} = 1 Osm
1 GEW (20 g) Ca^{++} = .5 Osm
1 mEq (20 mg) Ca^{++} = .5 mOsm
2 mEq (40 mg) Ca^{++} = 1 mOsm
1 mEq (35 mg) Cl^- = 1 mOsm

Therefore:

1 mEq (or .5 mOsm or 20 mg) Ca^{++} + 1 mEq (or 1 mOsm or 35 mg)
    Cl^- → 1 mEq (or 1.5 mOsm or 55 mg) $CaCl_2$

Remember:

1 mOsm of a monovalent ion = 1 mEq
1 mOsm of a bivalent ion = 2 mEq
.5 mOsm of a bivalent ion = 1 mEq

SOLUTIONS

There are many different kinds of solutions that are used routinely in the treatment of patients. Most of them are related to the GMW or GEW of the solute involved; 1 GMW of any solute is known as 1 mol or 1 mole of solute.

Molar Solutions

As its name would suggest, 1 molar solution contains 1 mole or 1 GMW of solute per liter of solution, or 1 millimole/ml of solution.

Example 1: dextrose, ($C_6H_{12}O_6$)

1 GMW or 1 mol of dextrose weighs 180 g. 1 GMW of dextrose per liter, or 1 Mol/L = 180 g/L or 18% D/W. Therefore, an 18% dextrose solution equals 1 molar dextrose solution.

The molar concentration of a solution is the number of mols or fraction of 1 mol of solute present in 1 L of solution. For example: 1 molar solution contains 1 GMW of solute/L; 4 molar solution contains 4 GMW of solute/L; 3.5 molar solution contains 3.5 GMW of solute/L; .3 molar solution contains .3 GMW of solute/L and; .15 molar solution contain .15 GMW of solute/L.

Therefore: 4 molar D/W contains 4(180 g) or 720 g of dextrose/L = 72% D/W; 3.5 molar D/W contains 3.5(180 g) or 630 g of dextrose/L = 63% D/W; .3 molar D/W contains .3(180 g) or 54 g/L = 5.4% D/W and; .15 molar D/W contains .15(180 g) or 27 g/L = 2.7% D/W.

Example 2: sodium chloride, (NaCl)

1 GMW or 1 mol of sodium chloride weighs 58 g. 1 GMW or 1 mol of NaCl/L = 58 g/L = 5.8% NaCl. Therefore, a 5.8% solution of NaCl equals 1 molar NaCl solution. 4 molar NaCl contains 4(58 g) or 232 g of NaCl/L = 23.2% NaCl. 3.5 molar NaCl contains 3.5(58 g) or

203 g of NaCl/L = 20.3% NaCl. .3 molar NaCl contains .3(58 g) or 17.4 g of NaCl/L = 1.74% NaCl. .15 molar NaCl contains .15(58 g) or 8.7 g of NaCl/L = .87% NaCl.

Example 3: calcium chloride, (CaCl$_2$)

1 GMW or 1 mol of calcium chloride weighs 110 g. 1 GMW or 1 mol of calcium chloride/L = 110 g/L = 11% CaCl$_2$ solution. Therefore, an 11% CaCl$_2$ solution equals 1 molar CaCl$_2$ solution. 4 molar CaCl$_2$ solution contains 4(110 g) or 440 g CaCl$_2$/L = 44% CaCl$_2$. 3.5 molar CaCl$_2$ solution contains 3.5(110 g) or 385 g CaCl$_2$/L = 38.5% CaCl$_2$. .3 molar CaCl$_2$ solution contains .3(110 g) or 33 g CaCl$_2$/L = 3.3% CaCl$_2$. .15 molar CaCl$_2$ solution contains .15(110 g) or 16.5 g CaCl$_2$/L = 1.65% CaCl$_2$.

Normal Solutions

In a 1 normal solution there is 1 GEW of solute/L of solution (1 mEq/ml); .5 normal solution contains .5 GEW of solute/L of solution (.5 mEq/ml).

Example 1: sodium chloride, (NaCl)

Because 1 GEW NaCl weighs 58 g 1 normal solution of NaCl contains 58 g/L.

$$58 \text{ g/L} = 5.8\% \text{ NaCl}$$

Therefore, 1 molar solution of NaCl equals 1 normal solution of NaCl and .5 molar solution of NaCl equals .5 normal solution of NaCl.

Example 2: calcium chloride, (CaCl$_2$)

Because 1 GEW CaCl$_2$ weighs 55 g 1 normal solution of CaCl$_2$ contains 55 g/L.

$$55 \text{ g/L} = 5.5\% \text{ CaCl}_2$$

Therefore, since CaCl$_2$ is a bivalent electrolyte, the concentration of a 1 normal solution is only half that of a 1 molar CaCl$_2$ solution; .5 molar CaCl$_2$ equals 1 normal CaCl$_2$.

Tonicity of Solutions

The tonicity of a solution refers to the degree of osmotic pressure exerted by the solution relative to that of body fluids.

Tonicity similar to that of body fluids is isotonic, iso-osmotic, or physiologic. (The prefix "iso" means "the same as.")
Tonicity greater than 300 mOsm/L is hypertonic, or hyperosmotic.
Tonicity less than 300 mOsm/L is hypotonic, or hypo-osmotic.

If the concentration of the plasma and interstitial Na$^+$ is hypertonic, or above normal, water will leave the tissue cells by osmosis to dilute the ECF. Water pushes itself into the interstitial fluid. The tissue cells shrink in size.

If the ECF Na$^+$ is hypotonic, or below normal, water will flow into the tissue cells by osmosis to dilute the fluid within the cell. The tissue cells swell.

Isotonic solutions given by a parenteral route neither increase nor decrease the size of any of the tissue cells.

Osmolality of Various Solutions

The osmolality of a solution is calculated by counting the number of solute particles in a given volume of solution; all the molecules of non-ionizing, nondiffusible solutes are added to all the nondiffusible ions of electrolytes existing in that solution.

1 GMW, or 1 Mol, of a non-ionizing solute equals 1 Osm.

1 GMW, or 1 Mol, or 1 GEW of a monovalent, ionizing, solute equals 2 Osm.

1 GMW, or 1 Mol, of a bivalent, ionizing solute equals 3 Osm.

The osmolality of a 1 molar, non-ionizing solution (which contains 1 Mol of solute/L) equals 1 Osm/L, or 1,000 mOsm/L.

The osmolality of a .3 molar, non-ionizing solution (which contains .3 Mol of solute/L) equals .3 osm/L, or 300 mOsm/L.

Example 1

What is the osmolality of 5.4% D/W? What is its tonicity? Since 5.4% D/W contains 54 g/L, and since 1 molar D/W is equal to 180 g/L the molarity of 5.4% D/W equals 54 g/L ÷ 180 g/Mol.

$$\frac{54 \cancel{g}}{L} \times \frac{Mol}{180 \cancel{g}} = .3 \text{ Mol/L or .3 molar solution of dextrose}$$

Since 1 molar dextrose solution equals 1 osmolar dextrose solution the osmolality of 5.4% D/W equals .3 molar or .3 osmolar or 300 mOsm/L. Therefore, 5.4% D/W is an isotonic solution.

Example 2

What is the osmolality of 50% D/W? What is its tonicity? Since 50% D/W contains 500 g/L, and since 1 molar D/W contains 180 g/L, the molarity of 50% D/W equals 500 g/L ÷ 180 g/Mol.

$$\frac{500 \cancel{g}}{L} \times \frac{Mol}{180 \cancel{g}} = 2.8 \text{ Mol/L or 2.8 molar solution of dextrose}$$

Since 1 molar D/W equals 1 osmolar D/W the osmolality of 50% D/W equals 2.8 molar, or 2.8 osmolar, or 2800 mOsm/L. Therefore, 50% D/W is a very hypertonic solution.

This example proves that 50% D/W is almost ten times as concentrated as normal body fluids. For this reason, 50% D/W is known as an osmotic diuretic. After intravenous injection, fluid goes into the blood from the ISF by osmosis, and is subsequently excreted by the kidneys.

Example 3

What is the osmolality of 5.4% NaCl? What is its tonicity? Since 5.4% NaCl equals 54 g/L, and since 1 molar NaCl contains 58 g/L the molarity of 5.4% NaCl equals 54 g/L ÷ 58 g/Mol.

$$\frac{54 \text{ g}}{L} \times \frac{Mol}{58 \text{ g}} = .93 \text{ Mol/L or } .93 \text{ molar NaCl solution}$$

Since 1 molar NaCl equals 2 osmolar NaCl the osmolality of 5.4% NaCl equals .93 molar NaCl × 2 = 1.86 osmolar, or 1860 mOsm/L. Therefore, 5.4% NaCl is a very hypertonic solution.

Example 4

What % NaCl solution will contain 300 mOsm/L? What % is isotonic?

$$300 \text{ mOsm/L} = .3 \text{ Osm/L}$$

$$1 \text{ Molar NaCl} = 2 \text{ Osm/L} = 2 \text{ Osm/Mol}$$

Therefore, the molarity of isotonic saline equals

$$.3 \text{ Osm/L} \div 2 \text{ Osm/Mol}$$

$$\frac{.3 \text{ Osm}}{L} \times \frac{Mol}{2 \text{ Osm}} = .15 \text{ Mol/L}$$

$$\% \text{ NaCl containing } 300 \text{ mOsm/L} = \frac{.15 \text{ Mol}}{L} \times \frac{58 \text{ g}}{Mol}$$

$$= 8.7 \text{ g/L} = .87\% \text{ NaCl solution}$$

A solution of NaCl that contains 300 mOsm/L = 8.7 g/L, or .87% NaCl.

Note: An error that medical personnel often make is to refer to physiologic or isotonic NaCl solutions as "normal saline." 1 normal saline contains 1 GEW NaCl/L. 1 GEW NaCl/L equals 58 g/L or 5.8%. Isotonic NaCl contains only 8.7 g of NaCl/L, which is a .15 molar solution of NaCl. .15 molar NaCl = .15 × 58 g/L = 8.7 g/L = .87% solution of NaCl.

Example 5

What is the osmolality of a 5.4% $CaCl_2$ solution? What is its tonicity? Since 5.4% $CaCl_2$ equals 54 g/L, and since 1 molar $CaCl_2$ solution equals 110 g/L, the molarity of 5.4% $CaCl_2$ equals 54 g/L ÷ 110 g/Mol.

$$\frac{54 \text{ g}}{L} \times \frac{Mol}{110 \text{ g}} = .49 \text{ Mol/L or } .49 \text{ molar } CaCl_2 \text{ solution}$$

Since the osmolality of 1 molar bivalent electrolyte solution is 3 Osm/L, and since 1 molar $CaCl_2$ solution equals 3 osmolar $CaCl_2$ solution:

osmolality of 5.4% $CaCl_2$ = .49 molar $CaCl_2 \times 3$

$$= 1.47 \text{ Osm/L, or } 1470 \text{ mOsm/L}$$

Therefore, 5.4% $CaCl_2$ is a very hypertonic solution.

Example 6

What % $CaCl_2$ solution will contain 300 mOsm/L, or is isotonic? 1 molar $CaCl_2$ = 3 Osm/L = 3 Osm/Mol. Therefore, the molarity of isotonic $CaCl_2$ solution =

$$\overset{.1}{\underset{}{\frac{.3 \text{ Osm}}{L}}} \times \frac{Mol}{3 \text{ Osm}} = \frac{.1 \text{ Mol}}{L}$$

.3 Osm/L ÷ 3 Osm/Mol

% $CaCl_2$ containing 300 mOsm/L =

$$\frac{.1 \text{ Mol}}{L} \times \frac{110 \text{ g}}{Mol} = 11.0 \text{ g/L} = 1.1\% \ CaCl_2 \text{ solution}$$

A solution of $CaCl_2$ that contains 300 mOsm/L equals 11 g/L, or 1.1%, which is isotonic $CaCl_2$.

Example 7

What is the mOsm concentration of .9% NaCl? The molar concentration of .9% NaCl equals 9 g/L ÷ 58 g/GMW of NaCl.

$$\frac{9 \text{ g}}{L} \times \frac{GMW}{58 \text{ g}} = \frac{.155 \text{ GMW}}{L} = .155 \text{ molar solution}$$

mOsm concentration/L of .9% NaCl equals

$$\frac{.155 \text{ Mol}}{L} \times \frac{2000 \text{ mOsm}}{Mol} = 310 \text{ mOsm/L}$$

Note: Physiological saline is manufactured as .85%, .87%, and .9% solutions. The mOsm concentration of all three of these solutions is considered to be isotonic.

Avogadro's Law and Solutions

Avogadro's law states that equal volumes of solutions of equal molarity contain the same number of Mols (GMW), and equal numbers of molecules. Avogadro's law is illustrated in Table 10.2. The table shows that ionizing solutions such as NaCl and $CaCl_2$ contain many more particles that exert osmotic pressure than do non-ionizing solutions such as glucose.

Table 10.2   Avogadro's Law and Solutions

Equal volumes of solutions of equal molarity contain the same number of mols (GMW), and equal number of molecules (Avogadro's law).

NaCl		Glucose
1 L water 1 GMW 1 mol NaCl	1 molar solutions	1 L water 1 GMW 1 mol Glucose
Volume (1 L)	=	Volume (1 L)
1 GMW (1 mol)	=	1 GMW (1 mol)
58 g/L	≠*	180 g/L
5.8% (5.8 g/100 ml)	≠	18% (18 g/100 ml)
6.02×10^{23} molecules	=	6.02×10^{23} molecules
12.04×10^{23} ions or particles	≠	Does not ionize

$CaCl_2$		Glucose
1 L water .5 GMW .5 mol $CaCl_2$	.5 molar solutions	1 L water .5 GMW .5 mol Glucose
Volume (1 L)	=	Volume (1 L)
.5 GMW (.5 mol)	=	.5 GMW (.5 mol)
55 g/L	≠	90 g/L
5.5%	≠	9.0%
3.01×10^{23} molecules	=	3.01×10^{23} molecules
9.03×10^{23} ions or particles	≠	Does not ionize

* does not equal

REVIEW PROBLEMS

Problem 1

The label on a Ringer's lactate bottle can be used to calculate its osmolality. The osmolality of Ringer's lactate can then be compared with the total mEq content of Ringer's lactate proved in Chap. 9, pp. 100–103.

The label on a 1,000-ml bottle of Ringer's lactate reads:

Ringer's Lactate

1,000-ml size

Each 100 ml contains:		Each 1,000 ml contains:			
		Cations:		Anions:	
NaCl	600 mg	Na⁺	130 mEq	Cl⁻	109 mEq
Na Lactate	310 mg	K⁺	4 mEq	Lactate⁻	28 mEq
$Na(C_3H_5O_3)$					
KCl	30 mg	Ca⁺⁺	3 mEq		
CaCl₂	20 mg				
	Totals:		137 mEq		137 mEq

Step 1   NaCl equals 600 mg/100 ml equals 6 g/L of Ringer's lactate. The molar concentration of 6 g/L of NaCl equals 6 g/L ÷ 58 g/GMW of NaCl

$$\frac{6\ \cancel{g}}{L} \times \frac{GMW}{58\ \cancel{g}} = .103\ GMW/L = .103\ Mol/L$$

Osmolality of 1 molar monovalent electrolyte solution = 2 Osm/Mol or 2000 mOsm/Mol. Therefore, the osmolality of 6 g/L NaCl is equal to:

$$\frac{.103\ \cancel{Mol}}{L} \times \frac{2,000\ mOsm}{\cancel{Mol}} = 206\ mOsm/L\ of\ Ringer's\ lactate$$

Step 2 $Na(C_3H_5O_3)$ = 310 mg/100 ml = 3.1 g/L of Ringer's lactate. The molar concentration of 3.1 g/L of $Na(C_3H_5O_3)$ =

$$3.1\ g/L \div 112\ g/GMW = \frac{3.1\ \cancel{g}}{L} \times \frac{GMW}{112\ \cancel{g}}$$

$$= .028\ GMW/L = .028\ Mol/L$$

Osmolality of 1 molar monovalent electrolyte solution is equal to 2 Osm/Mol. Therefore:

$$osmolality\ of\ 3.1\ g/L\ of\ Na\ lactate = \frac{.028\ \cancel{Mol}}{L} \times \frac{2,000\ mOsm}{\cancel{Mol}}$$

$$= 56\ mOsm/L\ of\ Ringer's\ lactate$$

Step 3

KCl = 30 mg/100 ml = .030 g/100 ml = .3 g/L of Ringer's lactate

Molar concentration of .3 g/L of KCl

$$= .3\ g/L \div 74\ g/GMW\ of\ KCl = .3\ \cancel{g}/L \times \frac{GMW}{74\ \cancel{g}}$$

$$= .004\ GMW/L = .004\ Mol/L$$

Osmolality of 1 molar monovalent electrolyte solution is 2,000 mOsm/ Mol. Therefore:

$$\text{osmolality of .3 g/L KCl} = \frac{.004 \ \cancel{\text{Mol}}}{L} \times \frac{2,000 \ \text{mOsm}}{\cancel{\text{Mol}}}$$

$$= 8 \ \text{mOsm/L of Ringer's lactate}$$

Step 4

$$CaCl_2 = 20 \ \text{mg}/100 \ \text{ml} = .020 \ \text{g}/100 \ \text{ml} = .2 \ \text{g/L of Ringer's lactate}$$

$$\text{molar concentration of .2 g/L of } CaCl_2 = \frac{.2 \ \text{g}}{L} \div \frac{110 \ \text{g}}{\text{GMW } CaCl_2}$$

$$= \frac{.2 \ \cancel{\text{g}}}{L} \times \frac{\text{GMW}}{110 \ \cancel{\text{g}}}$$

$$= \frac{.0018 \ \text{GMW}}{L} = \frac{.0018 \ \text{Mol}}{L}$$

Osmolality of 1 molar bivalent electrolyte solution = 3 Osm/Mol. Therefore:

$$\text{osmolality of .2 g/L of } CaCl_2 = \frac{.0018 \ \cancel{\text{Mol}}}{L} \times \frac{3,000 \ \text{mOsm}}{\cancel{\text{Mol}}}$$

$$= 5.4 \ \text{mOsm/L of Ringer's lactate}$$

Step 5   Total the mOsm concentration of all the components of the 1,000-ml bottle of Ringer's lactate. Since it is a physiologic solution, the total should be close to 300 mOsm/L.

	mOsm/L
NaCl	206
Na lactate	56
KCl	8
CaCl₂	5.4
	275.4 mOsm/L of Ringer's lactate

A solution containing 275 mOsm/L is considered to be physiologic.

Step 6   The osmolality of each substance in the bottle of Ringer's lactate is compared with its mEq content in Table 10.3. For review, it is suggested that the student recalculate all the figures in Table 10.3 to prove that they are correct (See Chap. 9, Problem 5, Steps 1—6.)

Table 10.3 Comparison of Osmolality and mEq Content of Ringer's Lactate, 1,000 ml

	Cations						Anions			
	mEq Na+	mOsm Na+	mEq K+	mOsm K+	mEq Ca++	mOsm Ca++	mEq Cl-	mOsm Cl-	mEq Lactate-	mOsm Lactate-
NaCl	103	103					103	103		
Na Lactate	28	28							28	28
KCl			4	4			4	4		
CaCl$_2$					3.6	1.8	3.6	3.6		
Totals	131 mEq	131 mOsm	4 mEq	4 mOsm	3.6 mEq	1.8 mOsm	110.6 mEq	110.6 mOsm	28 mEq	28 mOsm

131 mEq Na+ + 4 mEq K+ + 3.6 mEq Ca++ = 138.6 mEq cations
110.6 mEq Cl- + 28 mEq Lactate- = 138.6 mEq anions
138.6 mEq cations combine with 138.6 mEq anions
Number of cations = Number of anions
131 mOsm Na+ + 4 mOsm K+ + 1.8 mOsm Ca++ + 110.6 mOsm Cl- + 28 mOsm Lactate- = 275.4 mOsm/L of Ringer's Lactate

Problem 2

The label on a 1,000-ml bottle of intravenous fluid reads:

$$3\tfrac{1}{3}\% \text{ Dextrose and } .3\% \text{ Saline}$$

1,000-ml size

Each 100 ml contains:	mEq/L
Dextrose 3.33 g	Na+ 51
NaCl .3 g	Cl− 51

Is this a physiologic solution? Prove the equivalents on the label.

Step 1

molar concentration of $3\tfrac{1}{3}\%$ dextrose = 3.33 g/100 ml = 33.3 g/L

$$33.3 \text{ g/L} \div 180 \text{ g/GMW} = \frac{33.3 \text{ g}}{L} \times \frac{GMW}{180 \text{ g}}$$

$$= .185 \text{ GMW/L} = .185 \text{ Mol/L}$$

The osmolality of 1 molar non-electrolyte solution is 1,000 mOsm/ Mol. Therefore:

$$\text{osmolality of 33.3 g/L of dextrose} = \frac{.185 \text{ Mol}}{L} \times \frac{1,000 \text{ mOsm}}{\text{Mol}}$$

$$= 185 \text{ mOsm of dextrose/L of solution}$$

Step 2

molar concentration of .3% NaCl = .3 g/100 ml = 3 g/L

$$3 \text{ g/L} \div 58 \text{ g/GMW} = \frac{3 \text{ g}}{L} \times \frac{GMW}{58 \text{ g}} = .052 \text{ GMW/L} = .052 \text{ Mol/L}$$

osmolality of 1 molar monovalent electrolyte solution = 2,000 mOsm/Mol

$$\frac{.052 \text{ Mol}}{L} \times \frac{2,000 \text{ mOsm}}{\text{Mol}} = 104 \text{ mOsm of NaCl/L of solution}$$

Step 3   Add the mOsm concentrations of all the components in the 1,000-ml bottle:

	mOsm/L
Dextrose	185
NaCl	104
Total	289 mOsm/L

A solution with a mOsm concentration of 289 mOsm/L is considered to be physiologic.

Step 4   Proof of the label. The label states that there are:

$$Na^+ \quad 51 \text{ mEq}$$

$$Cl^- \quad 51 \text{ mEq}$$

mEq/L = (mg% × 10)/mEq weight

.3% NaCl = 3 g/L = 3,000 mg/L

mEq/L = 3,000 mg/L ÷ 58 mg/mEq

$$= \frac{3,000 \text{ mg}}{L} \times \frac{\text{mEq}}{58 \text{ mg}} = 51.7 \text{ mEq NaCl/L}$$

The label is correct:

$$51 \text{ mEq Na}^+ + 51 \text{ mEq Cl}^- \rightarrow 51 \text{ mEq NaCl}$$

Chapter 11
CONCEPT OF pH

Another important mathematical entity is known as pH. The Danish biochemist Sorenson devised the pH scale in an attempt to simplify discussion of astronomical numbers of hydrogen ions.

The numbers of hydrogen ions must be counted since it is the *numbers* of free H^+ in a solution that determine its acidity; the more H^+ in a solution, the more acid it is. The pH scale measures the degree of acidity or alkalinity of a solution. Not only is the pH of the various body fluids important, but so is the pH of all the drugs and solutions used to treat patients. The range of acidity/alkalinity compatible with human life is very narrow.

The method of measuring the acidity or alkalinity of any solution is directly related to equivalent weights and to Avogadro's law.

Avogadro taught that there are 6.02×10^{23} molecules in 1 GMW of any substance, or 6.02×10^{23} atoms in 1 GAW of any element. (See Chap. 6, *Avogadro's Law and Number*.) Table 11.1 is a table of the powers of 10, which shows where Avogadro's number fits into this table. This gigantic figure represents 602 sextillion atoms (particles) in 1 GAW, or 1 GEW of hydrogen. Since there are 1,000 mEq in 1 GEW, there are "only" 6.02×10^{20} or 602 quintillion H^+ in 1 mEq of H^+, which also is shown in Table 11.1.

$$6.02 \times 10^{23} \div 1,000 = 6.02 \times 10^{20}$$

(See Appendix, *Multiplying and Dividing Decimal Fractions by Powers of 10*.)

Table 11.2 is a scale of the powers of decimal fractions, and Table 11.3 applies this scale to the numbers of particles involved in fractions of 1 GEW. A glance at Tables 11.2 and 11.3 might give the impression that infinitesimal numbers are involved, but such is not the case. Table 11.3 represents fractional parts of the huge number 6.02×10^{23}.

The hydrogen ion concentration of 1 L of a solution is commonly abbreviated $[H^+]$. This abbreviation will be used hereafter to represent the hydrogen ion concentration per liter of solutions being discussed.

Table 11.3 shows that:

$$1 \text{ nanoEq} = .000\ 000\ 001 \text{ Eq}$$

and that

$$40 \text{ nanoEq} = .000\ 000\ 040 \text{ Eq}$$

135

Table 11.1 Powers of Ten (Whole Numbers)

$$10 = 1. \times 10 = \text{ten}$$
$$100 = 1. \times 10^2 = 1 \text{ hundred}$$
$$1,000 = 1. \times 10^3 = 1 \text{ thousand}$$
$$1,000,000 = 1. \times 10^6 = 1 \text{ million}$$
$$1,000,000,000 = 1. \times 10^9 = 1 \text{ billion}$$
$$1,000,000,000,000 = 1. \times 10^{12} = 1 \text{ trillion}$$
$$1,000,000,000,000,000 = 1. \times 10^{15} = 1 \text{ quadrillion}$$
$$1,000,000,000,000,000,000 = 1. \times 10^{18} = 1 \text{ quintillion}$$
$$602,000,000,000,000,000,000 = 6.02 \times 10^{20} = 602 \text{ quintillion}$$
$$1,000,000,000,000,000,000,000 = 1. \times 10^{21} = 1 \text{ sextillion}$$
$$602,000,000,000,000,000,000,000 = 6.02 \times 10^{23} = 602 \text{ sextillion}$$
$$\text{(Avogadro's number)}$$
$$1,000,000,000,000,000,000,000,000 = 1. \times 10^{24} = 1 \text{ septillion}$$

Table 11.2 Scale of Powers of Decimal Fractions

1/1	= 1.0	= $1. \times 10^0$
1/10	= .1	= $1. \times 10^{-1}$
1/100	= .01	= $1. \times 10^{-2}$
1/1,000	= .001	= $1. \times 10^{-3}$
1/10,000	= .000 1	= $1. \times 10^{-4}$
1/100,000	= .000 01	= $1. \times 10^{-5}$
1/1,000,000	= .000 001	= $1. \times 10^{-6}$
1/10,000,000	= .000 000 1	= $1. \times 10^{-7}$
1/100,000,000	= .000 000 01	= $1. \times 10^{-8}$
1/1,000,000,000	= .000 000 001	= $1. \times 10^{-9}$
1/10,000,000,000	= .000 000 000 1	= $1. \times 10^{-10}$
1/100,000,000,000	= .000 000 000 01	= $1. \times 10^{-11}$
1/1,000,000,000,000	= .000 000 000 001	= $1. \times 10^{-12}$

Table 11.3 Numbers of Particles Involved in Fractions of 1 GEW

1,000	mEq (milliequivalent)	= 1.000 Eq	= $1. \times 10^0$ Eq
100	mEq	= .100 Eq	= $1. \times 10^{-1}$ Eq
10	mEq	= .010 Eq	= $1. \times 10^{-2}$ Eq
1	mEq	= .001 Eq	= $1. \times 10^{-3}$ Eq
100	μEq (microequivalent)	= .000 100 Eq	= $1. \times 10^{-4}$ Eq
10	μEq	= .000 010 Eq	= $1. \times 10^{-5}$ Eq
1	μEq	= .000 001 Eq	= $1. \times 10^{-6}$ Eq
100	nEq (nanoequivalent)	= .000 000 100 Eq	= $1. \times 10^{-7}$ Eq
40	nEq	= .000 000 040 Eq	= $4. \times 10^{-8}$ Eq
10	nEq	= .000 000 010 Eq	= $1. \times 10^{-8}$ Eq
1	nEq	= .000 000 001 Eq	= $1. \times 10^{-9}$ Eq

(The symbol μ means microequivalent; n means nanoequivalent, often abbreviated nanoEq to avoid confusion with mEq, the abbreviation for milliequivalent.)

The normal [H^+] in the blood is .000 000 040 Eq/L, or 40 nanoEq/L;

.000 000 040 Eq/L = 40 × 10^{-9} Eq/L, or

4 × 10^{-8} Eq/L.   (See Appendix, *Exponents of 10.*)

Just how many H^+ there are in 40 nanoEq can easily be calculated:

$$\begin{array}{r} 6.02 \times 10^{23} \text{ ions in 1 GEW of } H^+ \\ \times \quad 4 \times 10^{-8} \text{ GEW of } H^+/L \text{ of normal blood} \\ \hline 24.08 \times 10^{15} \ H^+/L \text{ of normal blood} \end{array}$$

(See Appendix, *Exponent Method of Multiplying by Powers of 10.*)

Normally there are about 24 quadrillion, 80 trillion H^+/L of blood—certainly not a small number! This is the reason why the [H^+] of blood is known as 40 nanoEq/L of blood, which is a small number only when compared with other substances that are measured in mEq/L.

Example

Compare 24.08 × 10^{15} H^+/L of blood with 142 mEq of Na^+/L of blood. (See Chap. 8, Table 8.1)

142 mEq = .142 Eq of Na^+/L of blood

$$\begin{array}{r} 6.02 \times 10^{23} \quad \text{ions/GEW of } Na^+ \\ \times .142 \quad\quad \text{Eq of } Na^+/L \text{ of blood} \\ \hline .85484 \times 10^{23} \ Na^+/L \text{ of blood, or} \\ 85{,}484{,}000{,}000{,}000{,}000{,}000{,}000 \ Na^+/L \text{ of blood} \end{array}$$

Thus it is proved that there are:

24,080,000,000,000,000 H^+/L of blood and

85,484,000,000,000,000,000,000 Na^+/L of blood

It can also be calculated that:

.85484 × 10^{23} ÷ 24.08 × 10^{15} = 3,550,000

These figures prove that there are 3,550,000 times as many Na^+ as H^+ in 1 L of normal blood. (See Appendix, *Exponent Method of Dividing by Powers of 10.*) An easier way to prove this fact would be:

.142 Eq Na^+ ÷ .000 000 04 Eq H^+

= 3,550,000 times as many Na^+ as H^+/L of blood.

EXPLANATION OF pH

The abbreviation pH means power of the hydrogen ion concentration. The pH is the power to which the number 10 must be raised to find the exact number of hydrogen ions that exist in a liter of a given solution. The pH of a solution is, therefore, an exponent of the number 10.

The pH of a solution is also a logarithm, because logarithms express powers of 10. A discussion of logarithms is beyond the scope of this text, but really is not necessary. It is enough to know that a log is the exponent indicating the power to which the fixed number 10 must be raised to produce a given number.

Therefore, the pH of a solution is derived by converting the entire value of [H$^+$] (the number of hydrogen ions in 1 L of that solution) to a single exponent of 10 by calculating its logarithm.

The logarithms (or exponents of 10) of the hydrogen ion concentrations of solutions involved in biochemistry will always be negative, because the number of H$^+$ being counted is a fraction of 1 Eq of H$^+$ (6.02 $\times$ 10^{23} H$^+$). For this reason, in order to avoid dealing with negative numbers, Sorenson arbitrarily elected to change the sign of the negative exponent to positive, and call it pH.

The pH of a solution can be expressed by any one of the following equations:

$$pH = - \log \text{ of the } [H^+]$$

$$pH = \log 1/[H^+]$$

$$pH = \log \text{ of the } [H^+] \text{ expressed as a positive number}$$

$$[H^+] = 1 \times 10^{-pH} \text{ Eq of } H^+/L$$

$$[H^+] = 1/10^{pH} \text{ Eq of } H^+/L$$

(Just as 1 $\times$ 10^{-2} = 1/10^2 = 1/100 = .01, equations 4 and 5 are equalities. See Appendix, *Exponents of 10*.)

Example: pH of pure water

The [H$^+$] of pure water is 1 $\times$ 10^{-7} Eq/L or .000 000 1 Eq/L. Using equation 1

$$pH = -\log \text{ of the } [H^+]$$

$$\log [.000\ 000\ 1] = -7$$

$$pH = -(-7)$$

$$pH \text{ of water} = +7$$

Using equation 2

$$pH = \log 1/[H^+]$$

$$pH \text{ of water} = \log 1/.000\ 000\ 1$$

$$= \log 10,000,000 = 7$$

$$pH \text{ of water} = +7$$

Using equation 3

$$pH = \log \text{ of } [H^+] \text{ expressed as a positive number}$$

$$\log .000\ 000\ 1 = -7$$

pH of water $= +7$

Using equation 4

$$[H^+] = 1 \times 10^{-pH} \text{ Eq/L}$$

$$[H^+] = 1 \times 10^{-7} \text{ Eq/L}$$

$$[H^+] = .000\ 000\ 1 \text{ Eq/L}$$

Using equation 5

$$[H^+] = \frac{1}{10^{pH}} \text{ Eq/L}$$

$$[H^+] = \frac{1}{10^{7}} \text{ Eq/L}$$

$$[H^+] = \frac{1}{10,000,000} \text{ Eq/L}$$

$$[H^+] = .000\ 000\ 1 \text{ Eq/L}$$

Water is neutral. This means that it is neither acidic nor basic because there are identical numbers of H^+ and $(OH)^-$ in water.

$$.000\ 000\ 1 \text{ Eq } H^+ + .000\ 000\ 1 \text{ Eq } (OH)^- \rightarrow .000\ 000\ 1 \text{ Eq } H(OH)$$

There are:

$$\left. \begin{array}{l} 1 \times 10^{-7} \text{ Eq of free } H^+ \\ 1 \times 10^{-7} \text{ Eq of free } (OH)^- \end{array} \right\} \text{ in 1 L of pure water}$$

All the rest of the H^+ and $(OH)^-$ are combined molecules of water and have no effect on the pH. This is the reason why water is such a poor electrolyte. Only one of about 550,000,000 water molecules ionizes at ordinary temperatures.

$$H(OH) \xleftarrow{\quad\rightarrow\quad} H^+ + (OH)^-$$

pH of Acids and Bases

The $[H^+]$ of an acid is greater than .000 000 1 Eq/L. Therefore, since the pH is, in reality, a negative number, the pH of acids is *always* less than 7. The $[H^+]$ of bases is less than .000 000 1 Eq/L, so the pH of bases is *always* more than 7. The $[H^+]$, or pH, of pure water, which is a neutral $+7$, is used as a standard for comparison with all other solutions. The degree of acidity or alkalinity is determined by the amount the $[H^+]$ varies above or below 1×10^{-7} Eq/L (pH 7).

Example 1

When a solution has more free H^+ or fewer free $(OH)^-$ than pure water it is acidic. If a solution has a $[H^+]$ of 9.3×10^{-5} (or .000093) Eq/L, it has a higher $[H^+]$ than pure water. Therefore, it is an acid solution.

Its pH is 4.03, a value less than 7, which signifies an acid solution.

Example 2

When a solution has a $[H^+]$ of 2.4×10^{-9} (or .000 000 002 4) Eq/L, it has a lower $[H^+]$ than pure water. Therefore, it is an alkaline solution.

Its pH is 8.6, a value more than 7, which signifies an alkaline solution.

Example 3: pH of blood

It was stated above that the normal $[H^+]$ of blood was .000 000 040 Eq/L, or 40 nanoEq/L, or $4. \times 10^{-8}$ Eq/L. To figure the pH of blood, the equations at the beginning of this chapter are used again.

Using equation 1

$$pH = -\log [H^+]$$
$$pH \text{ of blood} = -(\log .000\ 000\ 04)$$
$$\log .000\ 000\ 04 = -7.4$$
$$pH \text{ of blood} = -(-7.4)$$
$$pH \text{ of blood} = +7.4$$

Using equation 2

$$pH = \log 1/[H^+]$$
$$pH \text{ of blood} = \log 1/.000\ 000\ 04$$
$$pH \text{ of blood} = \log 25,000,000 = 7.4$$

Using equation 3

$$pH = \log [H^+] \text{ expressed as a positive number}$$
$$pH \text{ of blood} = \log .000\ 000\ 04 \text{ expressed as a positive number}$$
$$\log .000\ 000\ 04 = -7.4$$
$$pH \text{ of blood} = +7.4$$

Equations 4 and 5 prove that the pH of blood is +7.4. These two equations are really the same.

$$[H^+] = 1 \times 10^{-pH} \text{ Eq/L}$$

$$[H^+] = \frac{1}{10^{+pH}} \text{ Eq/L}$$

$$[H^+] \text{ of blood} = 1 \times 10^{-7.4} \text{ Eq/L} = .000\ 000\ 04 \text{ Eq/L}$$

$$[H^+] \text{ of blood} = \frac{1}{10^{7.4}} \text{ Eq/L} = \frac{1}{25,118,864} \text{ Eq/L}$$

$$[H^+] \text{ of blood} = .000\ 000\ 04 \text{ Eq/L}$$

Since the pH of blood is more than 7, the $[H^+]$ of blood is less than that of water, so blood is slightly alkaline.

Example 4: pH of solutions

What is the pH of the following normal solutions of HCl?

a)   1.0 normal HCl

$$[H^+] \text{ of 1.0 normal solution of HCl} = 1 \text{ Eq } H^+/L$$

$$pH = \log 1/[H^+]$$

$$pH \text{ of 1.0 normal solution of HCl} = \log 1/1.0 = 0$$

b)   .01 normal HCl

$$[H^+] \text{ of .01 normal HCl} = .01 \text{ Eq/L}$$

$$pH \text{ of .01 normal HCl} = \log 1/.01 = \log 100 = 2$$

The pH of .01 normal HCl = 2

c)   .000 001 normal HCl

$$[H^+] \text{ of .000 001 normal HCl} = .000\ 001 \text{ Eq/L}$$

$$pH \text{ of .000 001 normal HCl} = \log \frac{1}{.000\ 001} = \log 1,000,000 = 6$$

pH of .000 001 normal HCl = 6

Example 5: pH of hydroxide solutions

To calculate the pH of a hydroxide solution, it must be known that the $[H^+]$ multiplied by the hydroxyl radical concentration per liter, abbreviated $[(OH)^-]$, *always* equals 1×10^{-14}.

$$[H^+] \times [(OH)^-] = 1 \times 10^{-14}$$

Solving this equation:

$$[H^+] = (1 \times 10^{-14})/[(OH)^-]$$

What is the pH of .01 normal NaOH solution?

[(OH)⁻] of .01 normal NaOH = .01 Eq/L, or 1×10^{-2} Eq/L

$$[H^+] = \frac{1 \times 10^{-14}}{1 \times 10^{-2}} = 1 \times 10^{-12} \text{ Eq/L}$$

(See Appendix, *Exponent Method of Dividing by Powers of 10.*)

Using Equation 2

$$\text{pH of .01 normal NaOH} = \log \frac{1}{1 \times 10^{-12}} = \log 1 \times 10^{12} = 12$$

pH of .01 normal NaOH = 12

Example 6: hydroxide concentration of blood

$$[H^+] \times [(OH)^-] = 1 \times 10^{-14}$$

$$[(OH)^-] = \frac{1 \times 10^{-14}}{[H^+]}$$

$$[H^+] \text{ of blood} = 4 \times 10^{-8} \text{ Eq/L}$$

$$[(OH)^-] = \frac{1 \times 10^{-14}}{4 \times 10^{-8}} \text{ Eq/L}$$

$$[(OH)^-] = .25 \times 10^{-6} \text{ Eq/L}$$

$$[(OH)^-] = .000\ 000\ 25 \text{ Eq/L}$$

(See Appendix, *Exponent Method of Dividing by Powers of 10.*)

Proof

$$\begin{array}{r} .25 \times 10^{-6} \text{ Eq (OH)}^-/L \\ \times \quad 4 \times 10^{-8} \text{ Eq H}^+/L \\ \hline 1.00 \times 10^{-14} \end{array}$$

(See Appendix, *Exponent Method of Multiplying by Powers of 10.*)

Summary of pH Concept

1. The pH is an exponent of 10 used to express the $[H^+]$.
2. The pH is the log of the $[H^+]$ used as a positive number.
3. To derive pH, convert the entire value of the $[H^+]$ of a solution to a single exponent of 10 by calculating its logarithm. The logarithm will always be negative, so the sign is arbitrarily changed from negative to positive. Example:

$$[H^+] \text{ of pure water} = 1 \times 10^{-7} \text{ or } .000\ 000\ 1 \text{ Eq/L}$$

$$\log \text{ of } 1 \times 10^{-7} = -7$$

$$\text{pH of pure water} = +7$$

4. A pH of 7 indicates that the [H+] and the [(OH)−] are the same. A pH of 7 is a neutral solution of pure water, and is neither acidic nor basic.
5. $[H^+] \times [(OH)^-] = 1 \times 10^{-14}$
6. A *decrease* of 1.0 on the pH scale means that the [H+] has been *multiplied* by 10. An *increase* of 1.0 on the pH scale means that the [H+] has been *divided* by 10.
    a. If the pH of a solution is 5, the [H+] is 10 times greater than that of a solution with a pH of 6.
    b. If the pH of a solution is 5, the [H+] is 100 times more than that of a solution with a pH of 7.
    c. If the pH of a solution is 9, the [H+] is 100 times less than that of a solution with a pH of 7.

Notice in Table 11.4 that:

1. At a pH of 7, the [H+] and the [(OH)−] are the same. This is a neutral solution of pure water.
2. The [H+] multiplied by the [(OH)−] always gives 14 decimal places.

$$[H^+] \times [(OH)^-] = 1 \times 10^{-14}$$

3. A decrease of 1.0 on the pH scale means that the [H+] has been multiplied by 10, and conversely, an increase of 1.0 on the pH scale means that the [H+] has been divided by 10.

Table 11.4 pH Scale

	When:	
[H+] =	pH =	[(OH)−] =
1.0 GEW/L of free H+	0	.000 000 000 000 01 Eq/L
.1	1	.000 000 000 000 1
.01	2	.000 000 000 001
.001	3	.000 000 000 01
.000 1	4	.000 000 000 1
.000 01	5	.000 000 001
.000 001	6	.000 000 01
.000 000 1	7	.000 000 1
.000 000 04	7.4	.000 000 25
.000 000 01	8	.000 001
.000 000 001	9	.000 01
.000 000 000 1	10	.000 1
.000 000 000 01	11	.001
.000 000 000 001	12	.01
.000 000 000 000 1	13	.1
.000 000 000 000 01	14	1.0 GEW/L of free (OH)−

APPLICATION OF pH TO HUMAN LIFE

The extracellular fluid [H$^+$] compatible with human life is very narrow. As shown in Table 11.5, it encompasses pH values between 6.8 and 7.8, with a *normal* range of 7.35–7.45. Deviations from this range in either direction are signs of abnormalities or illnesses that cause acidemia or alkalemia. Extreme deviations are life threatening.

    The number of hydrogen ions involved in the pH range compatible with human life is shown in Table 11.6.

    Notice the relationships between the numbers of hydrogen ions in Table 11.6:

1. A solution with a pH of 6.8 contains 10 times as many H$^+$ as does a solution with a pH of 7.8.

Table 11.5   pH Scale and Human Life

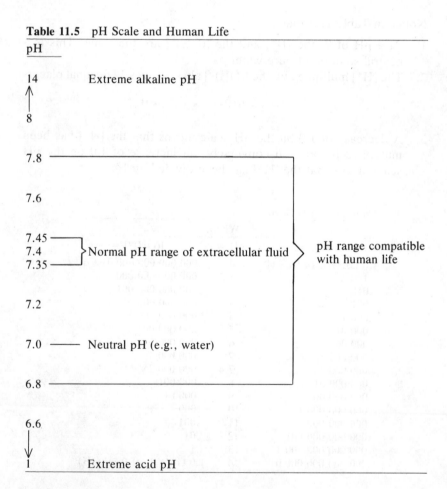

Table 11.6 pH and [H$^+$] Compatible With
Human Life

If the pH =	[H$^+$] =	or
6.8	.000 000 16 Eq/L	1.6 × 10^{-7} Eq/L
7.0	.000 000 1	1.0 × 10^{-7}
7.2	.000 000 063	6.3 × 10^{-8}
7.35	.000 000 044 6	4.46 × 10^{-8}
7.4	.000 000 04	4.0 × 10^{-8}
7.45	.000 000 035 4	3.54 × 10^{-8}
7.6	.000 000 025	2.5 × 10^{-8}
7.8	.000 000 016	1.6 × 10^{-8}
8.0	.000 000 01	1.0 × 10^{-8}

2. A pH of 7.0 contains 10 times as many H$^+$ as does a solution with a pH of 8.0.

3. A solution with a pH of 7.0 contains 2.5 times as many H$^+$ as does a solution with a pH of 7.4:

$$4 \times 10^{-8} \text{ Eq of H}^+ \text{ in 1 L of a solution with a pH of 7.4}$$
$$\underline{\times\ 2.5}$$
$$10.0 \times 10^{-8} \text{ Eq of H}^+ \text{ in 1 L of a solution with a pH of 7.0}$$
$$(10.0 \times 10^{-8} = 1 \times 10^{-7})$$

Compare these values with those recorded in Table 11.6. This example shows why a patient with a blood pH of 7 has a very serious acidemia (blood with high [H$^+$], or "acid" blood). He has an excess of 60 nanoEq H$^+$/L:

$$.000\ 000\ 100 \text{ Eq H}^+/\text{L of solution with a pH of 7.0}$$
$$\underline{-.000\ 000\ 040 \text{ Eq H}^+/\text{L of solution with a pH of 7.4}}$$
$$.000\ 000\ 060 \text{ Eq} \qquad \text{excess H}^+/\text{L of blood with a pH of 7.0}$$

The actual number of hydrogen ions in 60 nanoEq equals:

$$6.02 \times 10^{23} \text{ H}^+/\text{GEW}$$
$$\underline{\times\quad 6 \times 10^{-8} \text{ Eq}} \qquad \text{excess H}^+/\text{L of blood with a pH of 7.0}$$
$$36.12 \times 10^{15} \qquad \text{or } 3.612 \times 10^{16} \text{ excess H}^+/\text{L of blood with a pH}$$
$$\text{of 7.0}$$

60 nanoEq = 3.612 × 10^{16}, or 36,120,000,000,000,000 hydrogen ions!

Proof:

$$6.02 \times 10^{23} \text{ H}^+/\text{GEW}$$
$$\underline{\times\quad 1 \times 10^{-7} \text{ Eq H}^+/\text{L of solution with a pH of 7.0}}$$
$$6.02 \times 10^{16} \text{ H}^+/\text{L} \qquad \text{of solution with a pH of 7.0}$$

$$6.020 \times 10^{16} \text{ H}^+/\text{L of solution with a pH of 7.0}$$
$$\underline{-3.612 \times 10^{16} \text{ H}^+ \quad \text{in 60 nanoEq} \quad \text{(See Appendix, } Exponent\ Method}$$
$$of\ Adding\ and\ Subtracting\ by\ Powers\ of\ 10.)$$
$$2.408 \times 10^{16} \text{ H}^+/\text{L of solution with a pH of 7.4 (See p. 137, this chapter.)}$$

4. A solution with a pH of 7.8 contains .4 as many H^+ as does a solution with a pH of 7.4.

$$
\begin{array}{r}
.000\ 000\ 04 \text{ Eq } H^+/L \text{ of solution with a pH of 7.4} \\
\times \hspace{2.5cm} .4 \\
\hline
.000\ 000\ 016 \text{ Eq } H^+/L \text{ of solution with a pH of 7.8}
\end{array}
$$

Compare these values with those recorded in Table 11.6. This example shows why a patient with a blood pH of 7.8 has a very serious alkalemia (blood with low [H^+], or "alkaline" blood). He has a deficit of 24 nanoEq H^+/L of blood.

$$
\begin{array}{r}
.000\ 000\ 040 \text{ Eq of } H^+/L \text{ of solution with a pH of 7.4} \\
-.000\ 000\ 016 \text{ Eq of } H^+/L \text{ of solution with a pH of 7.8} \\
\hline
.000\ 000\ 024 \text{ Eq} \hspace{1.5cm} \text{deficit of } H^+/L \text{ of blood with a pH of 7.8}
\end{array}
$$

The actual number of hydrogen ions in 24 nanoEq is:

$$
\begin{array}{r}
6.02 \ \times 10^{23} \ H^+/GEW \\
\times\ 2.4 \ \times 10^{-8} \text{ Eq} \hspace{1cm} \text{deficit of } H^+/L \\
\hline
14.448 \times 10^{15} \hspace{1cm} \text{deficit of } H^+/L \text{ of blood with a pH of 7.8}
\end{array}
$$

24 nanoEq = 14,448,000,000,000,000 hydrogen ions

Proof:

$$
\begin{array}{r}
6.02 \ \times 10^{23} \ H^+/GEW \\
\times 1.6 \ \times 10^{-8} \text{ Eq} \hspace{1cm} \text{of } H^+/L \text{ of solution with a pH of 7.8} \\
\hline
9.632 \times 10^{15} \ H^+/L \hspace{1cm} \text{of solution with a pH of 7.8}
\end{array}
$$

$$
\begin{array}{r}
14.448 \times 10^{15} \text{ hydrogen ions in 24 nanoEq} \\
+\ 9.632 \times 10^{15} \text{ hydrogen ions/L of solution with a pH of 7.8}\quad \text{(See} \\
\text{Appendix, } \textit{Exponent Method of Adding and Subtracting} \\
\textit{by Powers of 10.)} \\
\hline
24.080 \times 10^{15} \text{ hydrogen ions/L of solution with a pH of 7.4}\quad \text{(See p.} \\
\text{137, this chapter.)}
\end{array}
$$

This example also shows that a solution with a pH of 7.4 contains 2.5 times as many hydrogen ions as does a solution with a pH of 7.8. This fact can be proven two ways:

a)

$$
\begin{array}{r}
1.6 \ \times 10^{-8} \text{ Eq of } H^+/L \text{ of solution with a pH of 7.8} \\
\times 2.5 \\
\hline
4.00 \times 10^{-8} \hspace{1cm} \text{or } .000\ 000\ 040 \text{ Eq of } H^+/L \text{ of solution with pH 7.4}
\end{array}
$$

b)

$$
\begin{array}{r}
9.632 \ \times 10^{15} \ H^+/L \text{ of solution with pH 7.8} \\
\times\ 2.5 \\
\hline
24.0800 \times 10^{15} \ H^+/L \text{ of solution with pH 7.4}
\end{array}
$$

An attempt has been made in this chapter to illustrate the astronomical numbers involved in the hydrogen ion concentration of various solutions, thereby demonstrating the need for the pH system to count them. The pH concept or pH notation as it is sometimes called is in wide use in science and medicine throughout the world today. If the mathematics behind its use is understood, pH can be a very useful tool. It is used as a part of blood gas interpretation, pulmonary function studies, respiratory care, and laboratory and other diagnostic studies. It is also an important consideration in the manufacture of drugs and solutions used in all fields of medicine and biological sciences.

Chapter 12
PRACTICE PROBLEMS IN THE MATH OF BIOCHEMISTRY

Refer to Table 6.1, Common GAW and Valences, in Chap. 6, p. 70 when necessary. Answers follow the problems.

1. Explain the following equality:

    $$20 \text{ mg } Ca^{++} = 39 \text{ mg } K^+$$

2. One mOsm of calcium = _____ mEq
3. On hand: 10-ml ampoule of $CaCl_2$, labeled "1 g in 10 ml."
    a. How many mEq of Ca^{++} are there in this ampoule?
    b. How many mEq of Cl^- are there in this ampoule?
    c. How many mEq of $CaCl_2$ are there in this ampoule?
    d. How many mOsm are there in the ampoule?
4. There are _____mg in 1 mEq H_2SO_4.
5. 1 mEq S^{--} = _____mg $(OH)^-$
6. 23 mg Na^+ = _____mEq Ca^{++}
7. 1 mEq Ca^{++} = _____mOsm
8. 1 mEq Ca^{++} + 1 mEq Cl^- = _____mEq $CaCl_2$
9. 1 mEq $CaCl_2$ _____mOsm
10. One GAW of S^{--} combines with 2 GAW of H^+ to make H_2S. What is the mEq weight of S^{--}?
11. On hand: 54 mg of HCl and a bottle of NaOH.
    a. How many mEq are in 54 mg of HCl?
    b. How much NaOH is needed for an exact reaction to take place?
    c. Write an equation showing the products formed and the number of mg of each reactant and each product. Prove it.
    d. How many mEq are there in each one of the products?
12. Define:
    a. Electrolyte
    b. Equivalent weight
    c. Milliequivalent weight

13. Define:
    a. Osmosis
    b. Osmotic pressure
14. Define:
    a. Osmol
    b. Milliosmol
    c. The osmolality of a solution
15. 1 mEq of a bivalent ion = _____mOsm.
16. Define:
    a. Molar solution
    b. Normal solution
    c. Physiological solution
17. Explain the difference between 1 normal NaCl solution and physiological saline.
18. Define:
    a. Hypertonic solution
    b. Hypotonic solution
    c. Isotonic, iso-osmotic, or physiological solution
19. The plasma proteins, to which the capillary membrane is impermeable, exert an osmotic pressure of about 25 mmHg. Why is this pressure important?
20. pH
    a. Define pH.
    b. If the pH of a solution is 8, the $[H^+]$ is _____ times _____ (more, less) than that of a solution with a pH of 6.
    c. If the pH of a solution is 7.2, it is more _____ (acid, alkaline) than that of a solution with a pH of 7.6.

ANSWERS

1. 1 mEq Ca^{++} = 1 mEq K^+
   Either one of them could replace 1 mEq H^+.
2. 2 mEq
3. a. 18.1 mEq
   b. 18.1 mEq
   c. 18.1 mEq
   d. 27.15 mOsm
4. 49 mg
5. 17 mg
6. 1 mEq
7. .5 mOsm
8. 1 mEq
9. 1.5 mOsm

10. 16 mg
11. a. 1.5 mEq
     b. 60 mg or 1.5 mEq
     c. 54 mg HCl + 60 mg NaOH → 27 mg HOH + 87 mg NaCl
         Proof:

$$54 + 60 = 27 + 87$$
$$114 = 114$$

     d. 1.5 mEq
12. a. Electrolyte:
         Substances whose molecules dissociate or split into ions
         when placed in water are electrolytes. Some develop positive
         charges and others negative charges.
     b. Equivalent weight:
         An equivalent weight is the unit of measure for the chemical
         combining activity of an electrolyte, dealing with the number
         of charges, not mass (gram weight). It is the chemical com-
         bining ability of the numbers of ions of any electrolyte that
         is equivalent to the combining ability of 1 GAW of H^+, which
         contains 6.02×10^{23} ions.
     c. 1 mEq = 1/1,000 Eq
13. a. Osmosis:
         A membrane used to separate two fluid compartments that
         is permeable to water or other solvent molecules but not to
         some of the dissolved solutes, is a semipermeable membrane.
         If the concentration of the nondiffusible solutes is greater on
         one side of the membrane than it is on the other, water
         molecules will pass through the semipermeable membrane
         toward the side with the greater concentration of nondiffu-
         sible solute. This process is known as osmosis.
     b. Osmotic pressure:
         That pressure in mmHg which, when applied to a solution,
         will just prevent the entrance of the solvent into it through
         a semipermeable membrane, is the osmotic pressure of that
         solution.
14. a. Osmol:
         An osmol is the unit of measure used to express osmotic
         pressure; 1 Osm = 6.02×10^{23} nondiffusible particles of
         solute.
     b. mOsm
         1 mOsm = 1/1,000 Osmol
     c. Osmolality of a solution:
         The osmolality of a solution is the number of Osm, or the

fraction of 1 Osm, dissolved in a given unit of solvent, usually
1 L. The osmolality of a solution is generally expressed as
Osm/L of solvent.

15. .5 mOsm
16. a. Molar solution:
       1 molar solution = 1 GMW/L
    b. Normal solution:
       1 normal solution = 1 GEW/L
    c. Physiological solution = 300 mOsm/L, the same as that of
       body fluids
17. One normal solution of NaCl contains 58 g of NaCl/L, which is
    a 5.8% solution. Physiological saline contains 8.7 g of NaCl/L,
    which is a .87% solution. It contains about 300 mOsm/L, the
    same as that of body fluids.
18. a. Hypertonic solution:
       A hypertonic solution is a solution that has a tonicity greater
       than 300 mOsm/L.
    b. Hypotonic solution:
       A hypotonic solution is a solution that has a tonicity less
       than 300 mOsm/L.
    c. Isotonic, iso-osmotic, or physiological solution:
       These terms are synonymous. Such a solution has a tonicity
       similar to that of body fluids (300 mOsm/L). The prefix "iso"
       means "the same as."
19. The plasma proteins create the osmotic pressure gradient that
    brings water and waste products by osmosis into the venous
    blood from the interstitial fluid. Without the plasma proteins,
    water and waste products would not diffuse by osmosis into the
    venous end of the capillary.
20. a. pH:
       The pH is an exponent of 10, used to express the $[H^+]$;
       It is a log $[H^+]$ expressed as a positive number. pH means
       the power of the $[H^+]$, and can be expressed by the equation:

$$[H^+] = 10^{-pH}$$

    b. 100 times less
    c. acid

SECTION THREE

STATISTICAL ANALYSIS

Chapter 13
FREQUENCY DISTRIBUTIONS, GRAPHS, PERCENTILES

It is not the objective of this section to give an extensive course in the calculation of statistical formulas to enable the reader to write a dissertation or research study; there are many excellent texts available devoted entirely to this subject. Rather, the intent is to present a simple discussion concerning the interpretation of the statistical statements, symbols, graphs, charts, etc. that are encountered in professional journals, periodicals, textbooks, and other printed matter.

Considering the enormous amount of printed matter available to the public, it is imperative that any medical science student be very selective about what he reads. In addition, every student must be very critical of the content of what he reads, recognizing that all to which he is exposed is not necessarily true. It is unfortunate that much of the current literature is biased, and that even statistics can be made to lie (Huff, 1954). For this reason, students in the medical sciences, especially, must be extremely cautious before incorporating new unsubstantiated data into clinical practice.

Statistics is "the math of the collection, organization, and interpretation of numerical data, especially the analysis of population characteristics by inference, from sampling" (Morris, 1969). Textbooks of statistical mathematics divide the subject into two fields: descriptive and inferential statistics. "*Descriptive statistics*" is precise because it states facts, for example the vital statistics printed in the newspapers about births, deaths, marriages, etc. They do not generalize or make predictions. Descriptive statistics collects and organizes facts only. If the entire population of cases in which one is interested can be observed, full information about observations made can then be summarized by descriptive statistical analysis.

Very often it is impossible or impractical to observe an entire population, so a representative sample of the population (sometimes called total or parent population) is drawn and studied, with the hope that the results of the study will apply to any individual in the population.

Whenever a random or representative sample of a population is drawn, the effect of chance causes a difference between the sample and the total population, but the larger the sample, the closer the sample actually represents the population. Results from studies of samples are used to predict the occurrences in the population. Such predictions, generalizations, estimations, etc., are known as *"inferential statistics."* It is inferred that an event will occur in the population because it was observed in the representative sample.

To make such inferences, attempts must first be made to justify them. A high probability that the inference is true must be mathematically proved from the observed sample data. This high probability is known as the *confidence level*. Biological sciences generally require that an inference be true in at least 95 out of 100 cases. Statistically this inference is expressed as "$p = .95$," where "p" means probability and ".95" means 95% of the time. A 95% confidence level means that 95% of the population will fall within a *confidence interval,* which is a band of values computed from the sample data. In other words, the "true" value of the unknown population must fall within this estimated band of values. It must always be remembered that although a 95% confidence level indicates that there are 95 chances in 100 that the population averages will fall within an estimated confidence interval, there also are 5 chances in 100 that the true population averages may actually fall outside the calculated confidence interval. When interpreting data, this fact should always be remembered.

In addition to a high probability that an inference is true, it must also be proved mathematically that the inference is reliable (tests that are repeated give the same results), and that the research method is valid (that it really tests what it claims to test).

A few common statistical symbols are listed below:

f	frequency, or number of times a score appears
N	number of scores, or cases
$\sum$ (capital sigma)	sum of
$\Sigma f = N$	the sum of the frequencies equals the number of cases or scores
x	one variable that expresses differences in magnitude Example: one exam on which there are many scores
X	one measurement on a variable Example: X is one score on exam x

p probability
H_0 null hypothesis
χ^2 chi-square

Some common mathematical expressions are:

$X = Y$ X equals Y
$X \neq Y$ X does not equal Y
$X > Y$ X is more than Y
$X < Y$ X is less than Y
$X \geq Y$ X is equal to or more than Y
$X \leq Y$ X is equal to or less than Y

Parameters are values that refer to parent or total populations. Examples of such populations are:

all first year medical students in the United States;
all the patients with cardiac insufficiency in University Hospital;
all teenagers in North America.

Values accumulated in a study of such populations are known as parameters.

Values accumulated in a study of samples of such populations are known as statistics. A few of them, and their statistical symbols, are shown below:

	Parameters	Statistics
Mean	m	$\overline{X}$
Standard deviation	σ	s
Number of cases or scores	n	N
Pearson correlation coefficient	R	r

At the risk of oversimplification, very simple figures are used to illustrate the use of various statistical symbols.

FREQUENCY DISTRIBUTIONS AND RANGE

Scores obtained by 30 medical students on an anatomy exam x are shown in Table 13.1. Such scores are known as raw scores.

The highest and the lowest raw scores found in Table 13.1 are 98 and 63. The statistical formula for the range of scores is:

highest score − lowest score + 1

The range of scores in this exam is:

$$98 - 63 + 1 = 36.$$

Table 13.1 Scores Obtained by 30 Medical
Students on Anatomy Exam *x*

63	72	93	79	72	73	
94	83	64	89	91	82	
93	87	74	77	71	76	$\Sigma\ X = 2433$
74	84	97	81	98	85	
79	85	82	78	78	79	

The range is used to determine the size of the intervals to be used in a frequency distribution. Table 13.2 is a frequency distribution representing the raw scores in Table 13.1. Since the range of raw scores is small, eight intervals of five scores each are used.

In Table 13.2, it can be seen that the sum of the frequencies is 30, which is the number of students who took the exam.

GRAPHS

Frequency Polygon

In all graphs, the vertical line is the Y axis (ordinate), and the horizontal line is the X axis (abscissa). Zero is the point where the X and Y meet. The frequency values are placed on the Y axis, and the test scores are placed on the X axis. Anatomy exam scores from the frequency distribution in Table 13.2 are illustrated in the frequency polygon in Figure 13.1.

Histogram

Figure 13.2 is a histogram that shows the anatomy exam scores from Table 13.2. If the midpoints of the top line of each of the columns in the histogram were connected, the same frequency polygon as Figure 13.1 would have been constructed.

Table 13.2 Frequency
Distribution For Raw Scores,
Anatomy Exam *x*, From Table 13.1

Score	Tally	*f* (frequency)
95–99	//	2
90–94	////	4
85–89	////	4
80–84	/////	5
75–79	///// //	7
70–74	///// /	6
65–69		0
60–64	//	2
		$\Sigma\ f = \overline{30}$

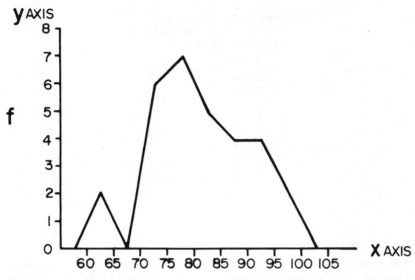

Figure 13.1.   Frequency Polygon of 30 Anatomy Exam, x, Scores from Table 13.2

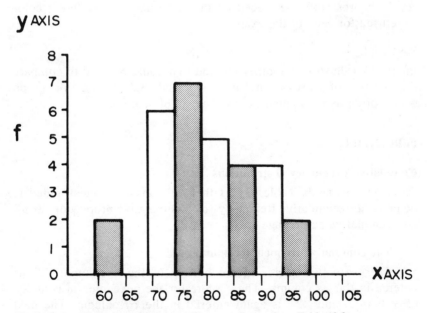

Figure 13.2.   Histogram of Anatomy Exam, x, Scores from Table 13.2

Table 13.3 Frequency
Distribution of Raw Scores,
Physiology Exam y

Score	f
95–99	0
90–94	3
85–89	3
80–84	5
75–79	8
70–74	4
65–69	4
60–64	3
	$\Sigma\, f = \overline{30}$

Bar Graph

A bar graph is an effective method used to compare two sets of scores. Table 13.3 is a frequency distribution of grades made on a physiology exam y by the same 30 medical students who took anatomy exam x (Table 13.2).

Figure 13.3 is a bar graph comparing scores made on anatomy exam x (from Table 13.2) with scores made on physiology exam y (from Table 13.3). An alternate type of bar graph comparing these two sets of scores could be placed on the same axes if a different color were used for each of the exams.

Pie Graph

Figure 13.4 illustrates another method that could be used to compare the two sets of scores from Tables 13.2 and 13.3. A single pie graph is also often used to illustrate just one set of scores.

PERCENTILES

Cumulative Frequency Distributions

Table 13.4 expands Table 13.2. Other columns have been added to demonstrate cumulative frequency (cf), cumulative proportions (cp), and cumulative percentage (cP).

The cumulative frequency column:

There are two scores at the bottom of the f column; "2" is entered in the cf column. The f score for the next interval is added ($2 + 0 = 2$) and "2" is again entered in the cf column. The next interval has six scores ($2 + 6 = 8$); 8 is recorded in the cf column.

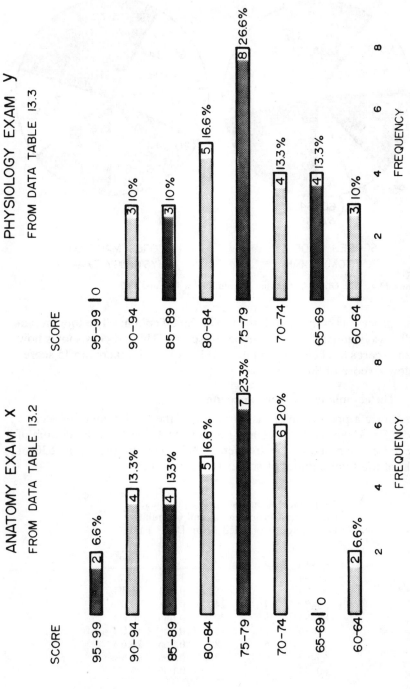

Figure 13.3.   Bar Graph Comparing Scores Made on Anatomy Exam x and Physiology Exam y

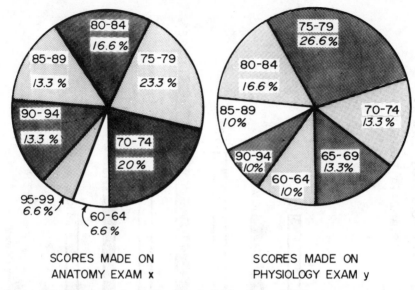

SCORES MADE ON
ANATOMY EXAM x

SCORES MADE ON
PHYSIOLOGY EXAM y

Figure 13.4. Pie Graph Comparing Data in Tables 13.2 and 13.3

This process is continued to the top of the cf column. The top interval will always equal the total number of scores. This process shows how many scores are below each interval. For example, there are 15 scores below a score of 80.

The cumulative proportion column

Since a proportion (p) is a fraction of the total number of scores, the cf is converted to a decimal fraction. In Table 13.4, the bottom of the cf column shows the frequency "2". This frequency is 2/30 or 1/15 of the total number of scores ($1 \div 15 = .066$).

Table 13.4 Cumulative Frequencies, Cumulative Proportions, and Cumulative Percentages Compiled From Data, Table 13.2

Score	f	cf	cp	cP
95–99	2	30	1.00	100%
90–94	4	28	0.933	93.3%
85–89	4	24	0.8	80.0%
80–84	5	20	0.666	66.6%
75–79	7	15	0.5	50.0%
70–74	6	8	0.266	26.6%
65–69	0	2	0.066	06.6%
60–64	2	2	0.066	06.6%

The next frequency in the cf column is 8. This frequency of 8 is 8/30 or 4/15 of the total number of scores (4/15 = .266). The rest of the column is filled in accordingly.

The cumulative percentage column

Previous practice with decimals and percentages in this text should make it easy to figure the cumulative percentage column. The decimals in the cumulative proportion column are multiplied by 100 to give the cumulative percentage.

Reading Centiles and Cumulative Percentage from the Ogive Curve

Data from the cumulative percentage column of Table 13.4 is plotted on Figure 13.5. Scores are indicated on the X axis, and cumulative percentage points are shown on the Y axis. The cumulative percentage curve, which is also known as an ogive curve, is drawn from these points. Any percentile point (often called centile point) can be read from a cumulative percentage or ogive curve. For example, the 25th percentile point is that point where 25% of the scores lie below it and 75% of the scores lie above it. Since 25% of the 30 scores is 7½ scores, it can be read in the cf column of Table 13.4 that 7½ scores fall in, or below, the 70–74 interval. This fact is shown by a heavy unbroken line in Figure 13.5.

The 50th percentile point is that point where 50% of the scores lie below it, and 50% of the scores lie above it. Since 50% of the 30 scores is 15 scores, it can be read in the cf column of Table 13.4 that 15 scores fall in or below the 75–79 interval. This fact is also shown by a heavy unbroken line in Figure 13.5. The 50th percentile point is also known as the *median*. (See below.)

The 75th percentile point lies within the 85–89 interval, a fact that is also illustrated in Figure 13.5. The 90th percentile point lies within the 90–94 interval. Any student who gets a score of 94 knows that more than 93% of his classmates scored below him. A student who gets a score of 74 knows that about 73% of his classmates did better than he did.

Naming the Most Common Percentiles

The 50th percentile is known as the median (Mdn) and is the middle point of all the scores.

Quartiles divide the distribution of scores into fourths:

The 25th percentile (centile) point (C25) is known as the first quartile (Q1), and is the point that separates the lowest quarter of the distribution from the upper three-quarters. (See Fig. 13.5.)

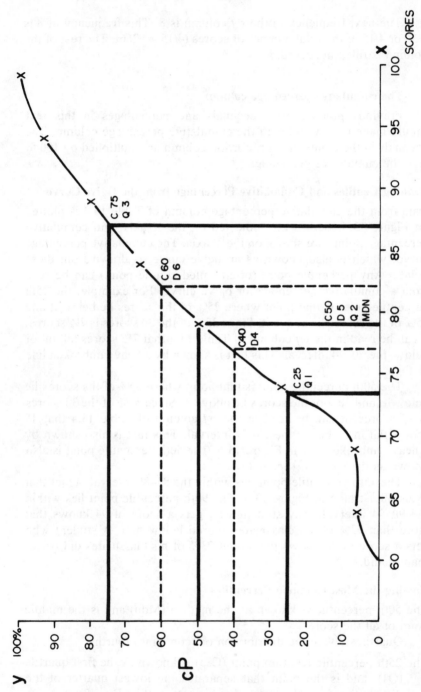

Figure 13.5. Cumulative Percentage or Ogive Curve for Data, Table 13.4

The 50th percentile point (C50) is known as the second quartile (Q2) as well as the median. Half the scores lie above and half below this point.

The 75th percentile point (C75) is the third quartile (Q3). One-fourth of the scores lie above and three-fourths of the scores lie below this point. (See Fig. 13.5.)

Deciles divide the distribution into ten equal parts. They have names similar to the centiles, progressing from low to high.

Decile 1 (D1) equals C10, or the 10th percentile point.

Decile 2 (D2) equals C20, or the 20th percentile point.

Decile 3 (D3) equals C30, or the 30th percentile point.

Decile 8 (D8) equals C80, or the 80th percentile point.

C50 = D5 = Q2 = Mdn

The 50th percentile (centile) point is the same as the fifth decile, which is the same as the second quartile, which is the same as the median. (See Fig. 13.5.)

Uses of Percentiles

Many exams such as National or State Board examinations or public school math, English, or science standardized tests, and various research data are reported in percentile ranks because of the ease of their interpretation. A student whose performance on an exam falls in the 67th percentile immediately knows he scored better than two-thirds of his classmates, but that one-third of them did better than he did. None the less, percentiles should be interpreted with caution. The percentile points fall very close together in the middle of a "normal" distribution (to be discussed in the next chapter). In Figure 13.5, compare the scores between C40 and C60 (black dotted lines). Notice that a change in only 5 or 6 raw score points (i.e., grades of about 77–82) corresponds to a change of 20 percentile units. Thus, the percentile reading in the middle of a distribution often has negligible meaning.

Chapter 14
MEASURES OF CENTRAL TENDENCY— STANDARD DEVIATION

There are three measures that describe groups of measurements or scores. They are known as measures of central tendency and are commonly called the mean, the median, and the mode.

The Mean ($\overline{X}$)

The mean is the arithmetical average of a group of scores or measurements. To figure the mean, all the individual scores X are added and this sum is divided by the number of scores N.

$$\overline{X} = \frac{\Sigma X}{N}$$

If the 30 scores from Table 13.1 are added:

$$\Sigma X = 2433$$

Since $N = 30$

$$\overline{X} = 2433/30 = 81.1$$

There are many other formulas for figuring the mean that are much easier when the figures get larger, but all that must be remembered is that the mean is the arithmetical average of the scores. The mean is used extensively in compiling other statistics because it is reliable and varies the least from sample to sample.

The Median (Mdn)

The median is the midpoint of a distribution. It indicates that point where 50% of the scores will lie above it, and 50% of them will lie below it. If there is a perfectly "normal" distribution (see "normal curves" below), the mean and the median are identical, but perfectly normal distributions are very rare. To approximate the median, the

167

number of scores is divided by 2. In Table 13.2 there are 30 scores; 50% or 1/2 of 30 scores is 15 scores (30 ÷ 2 = 15). The midpoint of the 30 scores lies between the 15th and the 16th scores; 50% of the scores will rank above this midpoint and 50% of them will rank below it. Exact formulas are available for figuring the median, but for the purposes of this text, "eyeballing" it in this manner is adequate.

The Mode (Mo)

The mode is the most frequently recurring score. In Table 13.4 the most frequently recurring score is 7, which lies in the 75–79 interval. The mode is most easily seen in Fig. 13.1 or 13.2.

Sometimes a set of scores has two or more intervals in which there are many scores. Such a situation is known as bimodal. For example: if five more students took the anatomy exam illustrated in Table 13.4, and all five of them scored in the 90–94 interval, f for that interval would then be 9. Both intervals 90–94 and 75–79 would then have a peak number of scores and the set of scores would be bimodal (See Fig. 14.4).

CURVES

Normal Curves (The Gaussian or Bell-shaped Curve)

A normal curve is a graph of a normal distribution. It has the greatest number of frequencies in the center of the graph, with smaller frequencies distributing themselves equally on both sides of the center line. Figure 14.1 shows that the mean, the median, and the mode are identical in a normal curve. Both Tables 13.2 and 13.3 contain scores that have produced reasonably normal curves.

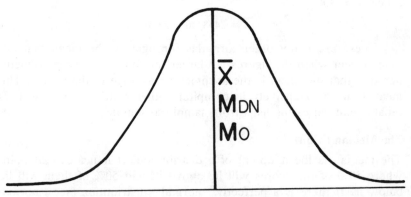

Figure 14.1. Normal Curve Showing that the Mean Score, the Median Score and the Mode Score are Identical

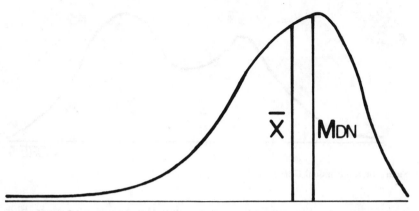

Figure 14.2. Negatively Skewed Curve Showing that the Mean Score is Lower than the Median Score

Skewed Curves

Sometimes the frequencies of a distribution tend to pile up on the left or right side of the curve, with long tails extending to the right or left. Such a curve is called a skewed curve.

A distribution is negatively skewed if the mean is less than the median and the tail is extended to the left. The negatively skewed curve in Figure 14.2 could represent the distribution of scores on a very easy examination. Scores are predominantly high, so the median (middle score) is higher than the mean (average score). One very low score profoundly lowers the mean, but has little effect on the median.

The positively skewed curve in Figure 14.3 could represent the distribution of scores on a very difficult exam. The scores are predom-

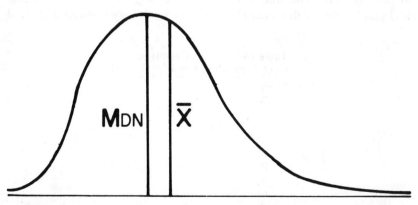

Figure 14.3. Positively Skewed Curve Showing that Median Score is Lower than the Mean Score

f

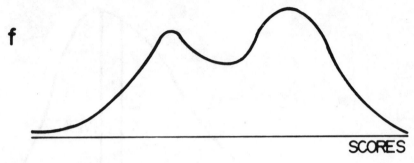

SCORES

Figure 14.4. Bimodal Curve

inantly low, so the median is lower than the mean. One very high score greatly affects the mean, but has little effect on the median.

Bimodal Curves

If a curve has two or more modes, it is said to be bimodal or multimodal. A graph of its distribution may look something like Figure 14.4.

Deceiving Aspects of Curves, and Measures of Central Tendency

In a normal distribution of scores, the mean, the median, and the mode are identical. Sometimes statistical data is presented with intentional bias, and the reader instinctively associates it with a normal curve. For example: ten people contributed the amounts indicated in Table 14.1 to a church building fund.

Can it truthfully be said that the average contribution in Table 14.1 is $121.50? Obviously this statement is misleading. To quote the median score, which is $10, would give a much more accurate account of the situation. The frequency polygon in Figure 14.5 shows Table 14.1 graphically. It demonstrates the very positively skewed data, and

Table 14.1 Contributions to Church Building Fund

$1000
100
50
10
10
10
10
10
10
5

$$\overline{\$1215} \div 10 = \overline{X} \text{ of } \$121.50$$

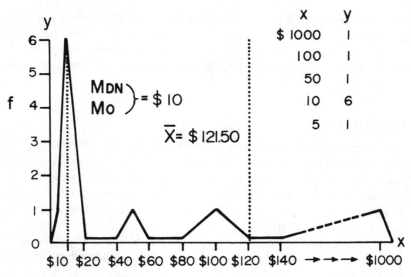

Figure 14.5. Frequency Polygon of Data, Table 14.1

shows how every measure in a distribution profoundly affects the mean. This is not so of the median. The top contribution could have been $1,000,000,000, but the median or mode would have still been $10. Notice how far the mean is deviated from the median in Figure 14.5. Situations when the use of the various measures of central tendency should be questioned are:

1. The mean, or arithmetical average, is deceptive when distributions are badly skewed. The extreme measurements profoundly affect the mean. As shown graphically in Figure 14.5, if a report states that the average donation was $121.50, the reader should ask, average of what data? What is the range; how many donors, etc.? The median is the best measure of central tendency for badly skewed data.
2. The median or middle point can also be misleading. Since the median is the 50th percentile point, the scores fall very close together in the middle of a normal distribution. As a result, the median is often meaningless.
3. The mode is seldom used except for the roughest and quickest estimate of central tendency. It is easy to compute at a glance, but it is very unstable.
4. The size or number in a sample is very important; only when there is a substantial number of trials or individual scores is the law of averages a useful tool. In addition, conditions need to be strin-

gently controlled to avoid bias. When analyzing data, notice the number of cases or scores involved. How many are enough? If a balanced dime is tossed 10 times, maybe 8 times it will come up heads, but if it is tossed 1,000 times, heads will come up about 500 times.

VARIABILITY

Variability is a term widely used in statistics. The mean, median, and mode are terms used to describe, respectively, the average, the middle point, and the most frequently recurring score. These measures of central tendency show where the center of the distribution is, but they do not indicate anything about how the individual scores deviate from that center of distribution.

In Table 13.1, the range of scores on anatomy exam x given to 30 medical students is 36. The lowest score is 63 and the highest score is 98. The mean score is 81.1.

Suppose the same exam were given to another group of 30 medical students, and the mean score of this group is also 81.1. However, the highest score is 88 and the lowest score is 72. Here the range is 88 − 72 + 1 = 17.

How can the differences between these two sets of scores be described? Both of them have the same mean score. This is done by measures of variability, which tell specifically how the individual raw scores disperse themselves around the mean score.

From the above example, it can be seen that the range of scores is a very unstable statistic. Just one score that is extremely high or extremely low can radically change the range. Table 14.1 shows a range of $996, but if the $1,000 contribution had not been included, the range would have been $96. This range is much closer to a normal distribution; however, it still would have been positively skewed to some degree. If the $100 contribution had also been omitted, the distribution would have been even closer to a normal one. Therefore, the range, like the mean, is used only in conjunction with other measures of variability, the most common of which is the standard deviation.

STANDARD DEVIATION

Unless all the scores or measurements are the same (i.e., each person in Table 14.1, for example, contributed exactly $10 to the building fund), some type of measure is needed to show the extent to which the scores are arranged around the mean (the average) score. The

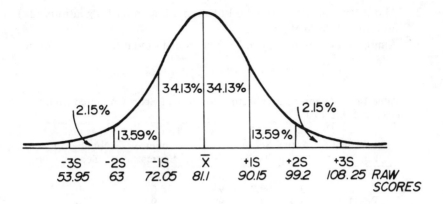

$\overline{X} \pm 3S$ INCLUDES 99.74% OF SCORES

$\overline{X} \pm 2S$ INCLUDES 95.44% OF SCORES

$\overline{X} \pm IS$ INCLUDES 68.26% OF SCORES

$S = 9.05$ (RAW SCORE POINTS)

$\overline{X} = 81.1$ (RAW SCORE POINTS)

Figure 14.6. Standard Deviation Units and the Normal Curve for Data, Table 13.2

standard deviation is the measure of variability designed to give this information at a glance.

When the scores of a set of data are plotted on a normal curve, the standard deviation units (s) are figured by a statistical formula found in any good text on statistical method. These standard deviation units are then measured off along the base line of the curve, starting from the mean and measuring in both directions into three intervals on each side of the mean. Those intervals to the right of the mean are positive, and those to the left are negative. If the curve is normal, these standard deviation units always cut off certain proportions of the area under the curve. Figure 14.6 shows the data taken from Table 13.2. The standard deviation units for this data have been calculated from a mathematical formula to equal 9.05 points, which is added to or subtracted from the mean (81.1) to represent the various standard deviation areas under the curve.

Figure 14.6 shows:

1. About two-thirds (68%) of the cases or scores in a normal distribution lie between ±1 standard deviation (1s) on either side of the mean.

2. About 95% of the scores lie between ±2 standard deviations (2s) on either side of the mean.
3. Almost no cases lie beyond ±3 standard deviations (3s) on either side of the mean.

Table 14.2 Theoretical vs Actual Number of Scores Adapted from Data in Table 13.1

Theoretical Limits	Actual Score Limits	%	Theoretical Number of Scores	Actual Number of Scores
$\overline{X} \pm 1s$	72.05– 90.15	68	20.47	21
$\overline{X} \pm 2s$	63 – 99.2	95	28.63	30
$\overline{X} \pm 3s$	53.95–108.25	99+	29.92	30
	$s = 9.05$ raw score points			

Note: Six standard deviations (3 on each side of the mean) cover the range of scores only when N is large, i.e., 500 scores or more. Here there are only 30 scores, so 4 deviations (2 on each side of the mean) include all of them.

Using the scores from Table 13.1 and data from Figure 14.6, Table 14.2 can easily be calculated.

Chapter 15
PROBABILITY, SAMPLING, AND STANDARD ERROR OF THE MEAN

A term used a great deal in statistics is hypothesis. A *hypothesis* is a premise that must be proved. It is an assumption or a proposition that leads to experimental research; data accumulated in the research is then reported to support or refute the hypothesis.

Example (greatly oversimplified)

Hypothesis: Drug X cures disease Y.
Experiment: Drug X is used on animals known to have disease Y. Detailed and accurate records are kept on the progress of the animals. The data accumulated is submitted to various statistical tests, and if the results of these tests prove to be statistically significant (see below), the data is reported in professional journals. When there is enough evidence that drug X not only is effective as a treatment for disease Y, but is also safe, approval for experimental use on humans is finally granted by the FDA.

PROBABILITY (p)

All experimental research involves probability of its truth (i.e., that the data presented is probably true), and a *probability statement* is included with all findings that are reported. There is always an element of uncertainty. The term probable is used in every-day conversation. The TV newscaster reports that it probably will rain tomorrow, or that there is a 60% chance that it will rain. Maybe the chance of a bad storm is so great that storm warnings or tornado warnings are posted. Rarely does the newscaster say that there is a 40% chance that it will not rain. This is implied.

If statistics show that a vaccination will prevent smallpox 99+% of the time, it is inferred that there is a remote chance that smallpox may develop, even if a person has been vaccinated. A doctor says that surgery will give the patient a 95% chance of being cured. The patient is not told that there is a 5% chance of death due to an inoperable disease.

In ordinary conversation, terms such as probably, possibly, or likely can be used without defining them exactly, but the terms always imply the chance that the event will *not* occur.

Chance is a tricky word. It means unexpected, random, or unpredictable events. It can be regarded as the probability that an event will occur if one takes a chance. Games of chance are a big risk to one's money, but there is a remote chance the player will win. There is a chance that a child may catch cold if he gets his feet wet.

Can statistics justify such statements? Scientists attempt to support or defend their findings by doing elaborate research studies. Then they make "scientific" guesses by using statistics computed from their accumulated data.

In statistics, probability values range from 1.00 to 0: 1.00 means 100% certainty that an event will occur; 0 means there is absolutely no chance that an event will occur.

Example

$p = 1.00$ that the sun will shine somewhere in the world today

$p = 0$ that an elephant will fly to the moon today

Most events have a probability somewhere between 0 and 1. If the weather forecaster says that there is only a 1% chance that it will rain tomorrow, he is also saying that $p = .01$ that it will rain, and implying that $p = .99$ that it will not rain.

What is the probability that a student can make a grade of 100 on a 25-item true-false test containing questions on material about which he knows absolutely nothing? Obviously, the probability is extremely low that he will guess well enough to get a grade of 100. Would he make a score of 0? Probably not, because chance would come into play and he would guess the right answer for some of the questions. A statistical formula can figure how many questions he would get right by chance alone.

If a statistic reads "$p = .01$", it means that there is a probability of only 1 in 100, or a 1% probability, that the information reported is caused by chance alone; $p = .05$ is a 5% chance; $p = .0005$ is a .05% chance, or 5 chances in 10,000 (1 in 2,000) that the outcome of the research is caused by chance alone.

When reporting medically related experiments, it is desired that the probability of chance be as low as possible.

Example

Extensive controlled studies have been done with drug X as a cure for disease Y. Results are very encouraging, because 88% of the patients with disease Y who were given drug X recovered completely as opposed to only 30% of the patients with disease Y who recovered spontaneously without the use of any drug. If the statistic states that $p = .01$, it is convincing because it means that there is only 1 chance in 100 that the results obtained in this study were due to chance alone. Drug X, therefore, must be effective in treating disease Y.

STATISTICAL SIGNIFICANCE

Probability is the degree of significance of research data. For example, $p = .05$ is a degree of significance placed upon research data. The *lower* p is, the more *statistically significant* the research data. The *higher* p is, the *less* significant the research.

SAMPLING

Inferential statistics report results of studies done on samples of populations, and make generalizations about populations based upon this data. Sweeping generalizations on any subject can be very dangerous:

Example

Fact: My mother makes good apple pie.
Fact: Your mother makes good apple pie. } = Sample

Generalization: Therefore, all mothers make good apple pie.} = Population

A generalization such as this would instantly be disclaimed, statistically, because it is based on an infinitesimal sampling of a huge population. This statement is ridiculous.

The technique of sampling populations, therefore, is an extremely important part of statistics, and detailed books and tables have been written just on this subject. It can be discussed only briefly here.

Random sampling is the very best and fairest type of sampling that can be done. A simple random sample is one where each individual in the population has an equal chance of being drawn into the sample. (The blind drawing of numbers from a spinning bin in a bingo game is true random sampling.) Random sampling is the only way that probability sampling should be done if statistical inference is to be made.

A random sample is said to be biased if every individual in the population does not have an equal chance to be drawn. For instance, if a random sample is taken for a study which states that "the population includes all United States citizens'' ignores those citizens living in Hawaii, the sample would be biased. To avoid this bias, the population should have been defined as ''all United States citizens living in continental U.S.A.,'' or else citizens living in Hawaii should also have been included in the sampling.

Finite Populations

If the population consists of a fixed number of units or persons, it is said to be finite. For example, a finite population could be 150 patients with fractured femurs in City Orthopedic Hospital. To study a sample of a finite population such as this, random sampling techniques should be used. A random sample of 15 of the 150 patients with fractured femurs, for instance, could be studied for the efficacy of a new type of surgery. Results of the study would be used for a comparison with results of traditional surgery performed on the remaining 135 patients, which are called the *control group*.

   If the entire finite population is to be studied, there is no problem with sampling. If all 150 patients with fractured femurs are included in the study, the results compiled from the study become descriptive statistics because no inferences are made. However, most often such a study would be used as a sampling of a population that included all patients treated for fractured femurs in the United States by a conventional method in the last ten years, for example. This population would be the *control group* with which the sample is compared.

Infinite Populations

If there is no limit to the number of units or persons in the population, it is said to be infinite. For example, an infinite population could be all the people in the world, all the stars in the universe, or all the people in the United States who ever had a fractured femur. If statistics compiled from a sample of such populations is to have any statistical significance, rigid random sampling techniques must be used. True random sampling is not easy. In medical studies the researcher is often limited in his sampling to the cases that happen to be available. He is forced to modify the random sampling rules by a specific or special sampling design that is appropriate for the study he wishes to do. Experience and judgment also often enter into the selection of samples in research in this nature, with the hope that statistical theory designed for random sampling will also apply to the study in question.

STANDARD ERROR

Standard error is a term used to tell how consistently, or accurately, a statistic measures. Never does any statistic measure any situation accurately 100% of the time. It may come close to this point, but never can reach it. The degree it deviates from 100% accuracy is known as standard error.

STANDARD ERROR OF THE MEAN ($s_{\bar{x}}$)

When studying very large populations, many samples are drawn in order to predict a norm or average. For example, if researchers wish to know the normal range of a hypothetical component of blood, called abc, that was recently discovered in adults in the United States, the following steps should be followed:

1. Blood is drawn from 50 randomly selected adults in each of 5,000 communities throughout the U.S. (one-third urban, one-third town, one-third rural, to avoid bias) and the concentration of abc/L of blood is determined for *each* individual in *each* sample.
2. The mean and standard deviation of *each* sample of 50 adults is computed. There will be 5,000 means and 5,000 standard deviations, each one representing 50 adults.
3. A frequency distribution of these 5,000 means is known as a *sampling distribution*.
4. The mean of this sampling distribution is computed and will be a good estimate of the population (or parameter) mean.
5. The variability (standard deviation) from the mean of the sampling distribution is the *standard error of the mean*, abbreviated $s_{\bar{x}}$. The standard error of the mean is important because it tells how much each sampling mean varies according to chance. When calculated by a statistical formula, the standard error of the mean of these samples is, in reality, the standard deviation of the sample means.
6. The actual mean and standard deviation of the abc content in blood of all adults in the United States is unknown. The mean of the 5,000 random sample means is used as an estimate of the mean of the parameter (abc in the blood of all adults in the United States) within a certain probability that the parameter mean will fall within a certain *confidence interval* (See below).

Example

The results of one group of 50 randomly selected healthy adults in the above hypothetical situation is shown in Table 15.1. The mean blood abc in this one sample was determined by formula to be 13.62 mg/L; the standard deviation is 1.05 mg/L. These results are shown under the normal curve A in Figure 15.1. Notice that the range of 99+% ($\pm 3s$) of the values in this one sample is 10.47–16.77 mg/L. In this one small sample of only 50 persons, all the values are included

Table 15.1   mg of abc/L Blood Drawn From
50 Healthy Adults in One Community

mg abc/L Blood	f	
15.5–15.9	2	
15.0–15.4	3	
14.5–14.9	6	
14.0–14.4	8	
13.5–13.9	10	$\bar{X} = 13.62$ mg/L
13.0–13.4	9	$s = 1.05$ mg/L
12.5–12.9	5	
12.0–12.4	4	
11.5–11.9	1	
11.0–11.4	2	
$\Sigma f = \overline{50}$		

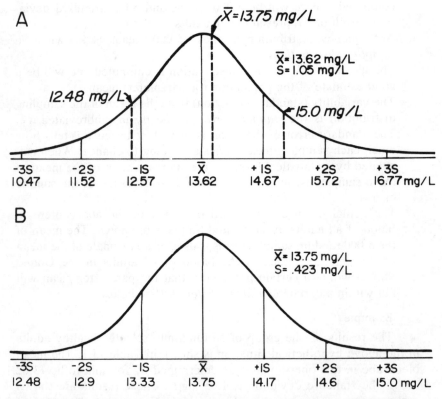

Figure 15.1.   Standard Error of the Mean from Sampling Distribution, Table 15.2 (B)
Superimposed on Standard Deviation Values Blood Sample Table 15.1 (A)

in less than $6s(\pm 3s)$. Only when there are at least 500 scores are $6s$ required to cover the entire range of scores.

The mean and standard deviation of each of the 5,000 samples of 50 adults are computed. There are 5,000 means and 5,000 standard deviations, each one representing the mean (average) mg of abc/L of blood from 50 adults. Table 15.2 is a frequency distribution of the means of 5,000 such samples. Such a frequency distribution is known as a *sampling distribution*.

The mean of this sampling distribution was computed by formula to be 13.75 mg of abc/L. This mean will be a good estimate of the unknown population mean (mg of abc/L in the blood of all adults in the United States).

The standard deviation of the means of this sampling distribution was calculated by formula to be .423 mg/L. It is known as the *standard error of the mean*.

The statistical results of the sampling distribution shown in Table 15.2 are illustrated under the normal curve B in Fig. 15.1. Notice how the range of $\pm 3s(12.48-15.0$ mg/L) under the B curve clusters around the mean in the A curve, indicated by dashed black lines. Also note that the means of the extreme scores of Table 15.2 (i.e., interval 15.0– 15.2, and most of intervals 12.0–12.5) lie outside or beyond $\pm 3s$. Thus it is demonstrated that when N is 500, about 6 standard deviations $(\pm 3s)$ include the entire range of scores. However, when N is 5,000, about 8 standard deviations $(\pm 4s)$ are needed to include all the scores. In this example $\pm 4s(12.058-15.442)$ includes all the scores in Table 15.2.

Obviously, the *smaller* the *standard error of the mean*, the more confident one can be that the results of a study are true estimates of

Table 15.2 Sampling Distribution of mg of abc/L
Blood From 5,000 Samples of 50 Persons Each

$\bar{X}$ mg abc/L Blood	f	
15.0–15.2	60	
14.7–14.9	65	
14.4–14.6	260	
14.1–14.3	440	
13.8–14.0	1,645	$\bar{X}$ = 13.75 mg/L
13.5–13.7	1,734	s = .423 mg/L
13.2–13.4	466	
12.9–13.1	205	
12.6–12.8	73	
12.3–12.5	32	
12.0–12.2	20	
	$\Sigma f = 5,000$	

the population values. The more samples taken and the more communities studied, the smaller the standard error of the mean will be, and the more reliable the estimate will be. This is true because the larger the sample, the closer it will truly represent the population.

Example

If the population is 500 persons, and the sample is 490 persons, the standard error of the mean will be extremely small. The sample results will be a very close estimate of the true values of the entire population. However, if the population is 200,000,000 persons, and the sample is only 10 persons, the standard error of the mean will be enormous, and the estimate of the values for the population will be worthless.

CONFIDENCE LEVELS AND INTERVALS

If $p = .05$ is the degree of significance claimed, most professional journals would write the statistic thus:

$$p < .05 \quad \text{or} \quad p \leq .05 \quad \text{or} \quad .05 > p > .01$$

These statistics translate, respectively:

p is less than .05;

p is less than or equal to .05;

.05 is more than p, which, in turn, is more than .01.

All of them indicate that the actual statistical point is within the interval between .05 and .01 values for p.

Example

From an appropriately large sampling for which a study is being done, a researcher reports:

$\bar{X}$ of the sampling distribution = 90 mg/L

$(p \leq .05)$ 90 mg $\pm$ 30 mg/L

This statistic informs the reader that there is a 95% certainty that the mean of the population will fall between 60 and 120 mg/L, which is a very wide range. This statement is not impressive for two reasons: the range is much too wide, and a 95% certainty generally is not good enough for medical studies. A 99% certainty is required as a rule.

Another journal reports:

$\bar{X}$ of the sampling distribution = 89.9 mg/L

$(p < .01) \pm .3$ mg/L

This is an impressive statement. It indicates that the sampling distribution mean (of an appropriately large sampling of the population for whatever the study) is 89.9 mg/L. The probability statement shows that there is less than 1 chance in 100 that the mean of the population will fall outside the narrow range of .6 mg/L (or 89.6–90.2 mg/L). Obviously this statistical report is much more reliable than the first one.

Many things can be predicted from the curve in Figure 15.1 B. It will be recalled that:

$\bar{X}$ of the sampling distribution in this study = 13.75 mg/L of blood

s = .423 mg/L of blood

1. The average person will have 13.75 mg/L of abc in his blood.
2. One can be 99% confident that healthy adults in the U.S. will have a mean blood abc that is within the range of 12.48–15.0 mg/L. Only one sample (of 50 persons) in 100 will have a mean blood abc that is outside this range of values. Since there are 5,000 samples in this study, it is to be expected that about 50 of them will lie outside this range of ± 3 standard errors of the mean. (Since "$p < .01$" means that less than 1 sample in 100 will lie outside the range of ± $3s_{\bar{x}}$, 50 samples (of 50 persons each) in 5,000 can be expected to fall beyond ± $3s_{\bar{x}}$.)
3. It can be stated that:

    $(p < .01)$ $\bar{X}$ blood abc = 13.75 ± 1.269 mg/L

    $(p < .01)$ is known as the *confidence level* for this study.

    The range of values stated at a certain confidence level is known as the *confidence interval*. In this example, in 99+% of the population (±3s), one can be confident that the mean blood abc will fall within the range of 13.75 ± 1.269 mg/L.
4. One can be 95+% confident that the mean blood abc of normal persons will be within the range of 12.9–14.6 mg/L (±2s). This statistic would be written:

    $(p < .05)$ $\bar{X}$ blood abc = 13.75 ± .846 mg/L.

    Meaning that: At a confidence level of $p < .05$, the mean blood abc will fall within the confidence interval of 12.9–14.6 mg/L.
5. The curve also indicates that one can be 68% confident ($\bar{X}$ ±1s) that the mean blood abc in healthy adults will fall within the confidence interval of 13.33–14.17 mg/L of blood.
6. Figure 15.1 B illustrates the very important fact that the more confident the researcher wants to be, the wider is the range of possibilities. If the degree of certainty (confidence level) is in-

creased from $p = .05$ to $p = .01$, the confidence interval becomes wider. The range of values that is being estimated becomes wider. In this example, one can be confident that 68% of the time the mean blood abc will fall within the narrow range of 13.33–14.17 mg/L, but 99% of the time he can only be certain that the mean blood abc will fall within the much wider range of 12.48–15.0 mg/L.

Chapter 16
STANDARD SCORES, THE NORMAL CURVE AND THE PEARSON *r*

Standard scores (also known as standard units or *z* scores) indicate how many standard deviations a raw score lies above or below the mean. A negative score signifies a raw score lower than the mean score, and a positive score indicates a raw score higher than the mean score.

z SCORES

A *z* score states the number of standard deviations a given raw score is from the mean score. The mean score and standard deviation are computed from a set of raw scores such as those in Table 13.1, which has a mean of 81.1 and a standard deviation of 9.05. The *z* score can be computed from the mean score and standard deviation, as shown in Table 16.1, and illustrated in Figure 16.1 (See also Fig. 14.6).

A *z* score is the raw score minus the mean score divided by the standard deviation.

Example

To figure the *z* score for a raw score of 94 taken from Table 13.1:

$$z \text{ score} = \frac{94 - 81.1}{9.05} = +1.43$$

A *z* score of +1.43 is almost 1½ standard deviations above the mean score. This is a very good score, as is indicated on Figure 16.1.

Example

To figure the *z* score for a raw score of 64, taken from Table 13.1:

$$z \text{ score} = \frac{64 - 81.1}{9.05} = -1.9$$

Table 16.1   Figuring z scores from Raw Scores, Table 13.1

z score		Raw Score
$0 = \overline{X}$	$= 81.1$	$= 81.1$
$+1 = \overline{X} + 1s$	$= 81.1 + 1(9.05)$	$= 90.15$
$+2 = \overline{X} + 2s$	$= 81.1 + 2(9.05)$	$= 99.2$
$+3 = \overline{X} + 3s$	$= 81.1 + 3(9.05)$	$= 108.25$
$-1 = \overline{X} - 1s$	$= 81.1 - 1(9.05)$	$= 72.05$
$-2 = \overline{X} - 2s$	$= 81.1 - 2(9.05)$	$= 63$
$-3 = \overline{X} - 3s$	$= 81.1 - 3(9.05)$	$= 53.95$

A z score of -1.9 is almost 2 standard deviations below the mean, and therefore is a very poor grade, as is indicated on Figure 16.1.

A z score of 0 indicates a raw score that lies exactly at the mean. Since 3 standard deviations on either side of the mean include almost 100% of the scores, it can be seen that the highest z score rarely exceeds $+3$, and the lowest z score is rarely less than -3. As shown on Figure 16.1, z scores have a mean of 0 and a standard deviation of 1.

OTHER STANDARD SCORES

Since handling negative figures is not easy, z scores are often changed to a larger scale, using all positive numbers. Negative scores are entirely eliminated, and by using a much larger standard deviation, all decimals can also be eliminated. This is easy to do by use of the following formula:

$$\text{Standard score} = z \text{ score (new } s) + \text{new mean}$$

T Scores (Also Known as Navy Scores)

T scores use a mean of 50 and a standard deviation of 10. By use of the above formula:

$$T \text{ score} = (z \text{ score} \times 10) + 50$$

To figure the T score for a z score of $+1.43$ that was calculated above:

$$T \text{ score} = (1.43 \times 10) + 50$$
$$= 14.3 + 50$$
$$= 64.3 \quad \text{(See Fig. 16.1.)}$$

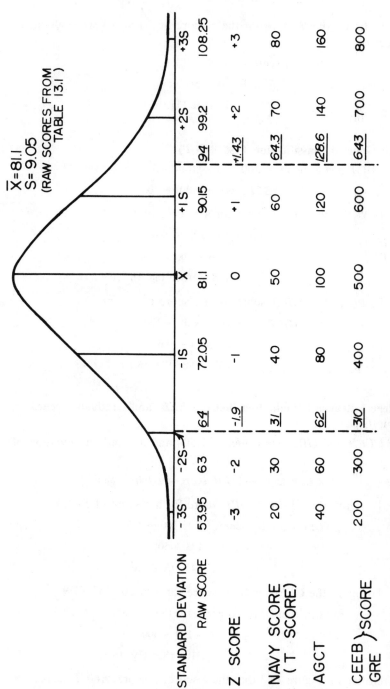

STANDARD DEVIATION	-3S	-2S		-1S	X̄	+1S		+2S	+3S
RAW SCORE	53.95	63	<u>64</u>	72.05	81.1	90.15	<u>94</u>	99.2	108.25
Z SCORE	-3	-2	<u>-1.9</u>	-1	0	+1	<u>+1.43</u>	+2	+3
NAVY SCORE (T SCORE)	20	30	<u>31</u>	40	50	60	<u>64.3</u>	70	80
AGCT	40	60	<u>62</u>	80	100	120	<u>128.6</u>	140	160
CEEB ⟩ SCORE GRE	200	300	<u>310</u>	400	500	600	<u>643</u>	700	800

$\bar{X} = 81.1$
$S = 9.05$
(RAW SCORES FROM TABLE 13.1)

Figure 16.1. Relation of Standard Scores to Standard Deviation

To figure the T score for the z score of -1.9 that was calculated above:

$$T \text{ score} = (-1.9 \times 10) + 50$$
$$= -19 + 50$$
$$= 31 \quad \text{(See Fig. 16.1.)}$$

Army General Classification Test (*AGCT*)

The *AGCT* has a mean of 100 and a standard deviation of 20.

$$AGCT \text{ score} = z(20) + 100$$

To figure the *AGCT* score for a z score of 1.43:

$$AGCT \text{ score} = 1.43(20) + 100$$
$$= 28.6 + 100$$
$$= 128.6 \quad \text{(See Fig. 16.1.)}$$

To figure the *AGCT* score for a z score of -1.9:

$$AGCT \text{ score} = -1.9(20) + 100$$
$$= -38.0 + 100$$
$$= 62 \quad \text{(See Fig. 16.1.)}$$

College Entrance Examination Board (*CEEB*) and Graduate Records Exam (*GRE*)

The *CEEB* and *GRE* use a mean of 500 and a standard deviation of 100.

$$CEEB \text{ score and } GRE \text{ score} = z(100) + 500$$

To figure the *CEEB* or *GRE* score for a z score of 1.43:

$$CEEB \text{ or } GRE \text{ score} = 1.43(100) + 500$$
$$= 143 + 500$$
$$= 643 \quad \text{(See Fig. 16.1.)}$$

To figure the *CEEB* or *GRE* score for a z score of -1.9:

$$CEEB \text{ or } GRE \text{ score} = -1.9(100) + 500$$
$$= -190 + 500$$
$$= 310 \quad \text{(See Fig. 16.1.)}$$

Notice on Figure 16.1 that the z score, T score, *AGCT* score, and *CEEB* or *GRE* score all rest at the same point under the curve.

CORRELATION

So far, how one score or measurement in a variable differs from all the other scores in that variable has been discussed. Now one group of scores or measurements can be compared with another group of scores. Correlation measures the relationship between two sets or groups of scores or variables. For simplicity, a comparison will be made between 10 of the scores made by the medical students in Tables 13.1 and 13.3 on the anatomy and physiology examinations. The raw scores made on the two examinations are recorded in Table 16.2.

A casual glance at Table 16.2 shows that on the whole, a student who did well in the anatomy exam also did well in the physiology exam, and one who did not do well in anatomy did not do well in physiology either.

THE PEARSON *r*

The statistic used most often to describe a relationship that exists between any two variables (sets of scores such as Table 16.2) is known as the *Pearson Product-Moment Correlation Coefficient,* abbreviated *r*. The *r* may vary in size from +1.00 through 0 to −1.00, and assumes a normal distribution of scores.

The Positive Pearson *r*

An *r* of +1.00 indicates a perfect positive relationship between two sets of scores. If each student in Table 16.2 made exactly the same grade in both exams, the two sets of scores would have a perfect positive relationship and *r* would equal +1.00. The *r* for Table 16.2

Table 16.2 Raw Scores Made By 10 Medical Students in Examinations *X* and *Y*, Adapted From Tables 13.1 and 13.3

Student	X (Anatomy Examination)	Y (Physiology Examination)
A	94	93
B	93	89
C	87	78
D	85	85
E	84	83
F	82	91
G	81	76
H	78	73
I	73	69
J	64	68

can be figured by statistical formula to equal +.84. This is a very high correlation and indicates that the scores made on these two tests tend to be associated, i.e., that students who did well in anatomy also did well in physiology, as was observed at a casual glance. However, just glancing at two sets of data rarely demonstrates any conclusive relationship. Therefore, this statistic must be calculated mathematically.

When interpreting experimental data presented in a professional journal, for example, one must be sure that the sample of the population is large enough. Here the sample is 10 of a population of 30 medical students, a very adequate percentage. But, if a sample of the grades of only two medical students had been used, the statistic produced would mean very little.

Figure 16.2 is a scattergram of the two sets of scores in Table 16.2. The broken straight line shows a perfect positive relationship, r = +1.00. Such a line would be created if, for every increase of one unit on the Y variable, there is a corresponding increase of one unit on the X variable.

Example

Suppose student A in Table 16.2 scored 94 on both examinations, student B scored 93 on both exams, student C scored 87 on both exams, etc. Although such a relationship would be extremely rare, it should be obvious that the closer the scores cluster around this straight line, the more closely related the two variables are, and the closer r approaches +1.00. Notice how the ellipse drawn around the raw scores in Fig. 16.2 follows the axis of the perfect positive straight line.

The relationship between the X and Y axes does not necessarily have to be on a one-to-one basis. The only requirement for correlation is that the relationship be consistent. If, for example, for every increase of two units on the X axis, there is an increase of only one unit on the Y axis, this too would be a perfect positive relationship.

The Negative Pearson r

An r of −1.00 indicates a perfect negative or inverse relationship between two variables. Sometimes a high score on one set of scores relates to low scores on a second set of scores. Suppose the physiology scores in Table 16.2 were exactly reversed. (Perhaps, similar to a golf game, low scores in this particular exam indicated the best result.) Table 16.3 records the exam scores from Table 16.2 with the physiology exam scores reversed.

The correlation of the raw scores for the two exams in Table 16.3 is not as obvious as it is in Table 16.2, though a close look shows that a student who made a high score in the anatomy exam generally made

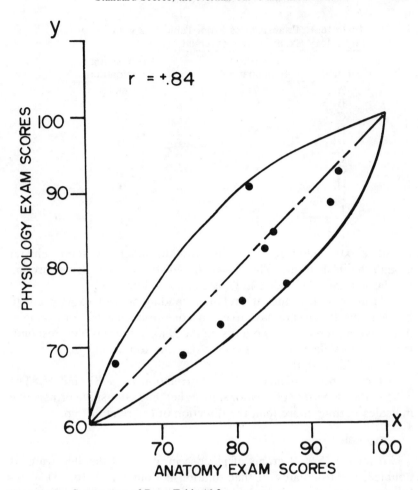

Figure 16.2.   Scattergram of Data, Table 16.2

a low score in the physiology exam. These scores have a correlation of $r = -.82$.

Figure 16.3 is a scattergram of the two sets of scores in Table 16.3. The dashed straight line shows a perfect negative relationship, or $r = -1.00$. Such a line would be created if, for every increase of one unit on the X variable, there is a corresponding decrease of one unit on the Y variable.

Example

If student A in Table 16.3 scored 94 in anatomy and 66 in physiology; student B, 93 and 67; student C, 87 and 73, etc., the relationship

Table 16.3   Exam Scores From Table 16.2 with
Physiology Exam Scores Reversed

Student	X(Anatomy Examination)	Y (Physiology Examination)
A	94	68
B	93	69
C	87	73
D	85	76
E	84	91
F	82	83
G	81	85
H	78	78
I	73	89
J	64	93

would be extremely rare. Notice the way the actual raw scores cluster around the dashed line. The closer they distribute themselves around the dashed line, the higher the correlation will be.

Again, only the student's relative standing on each exam needs to be the same. It does not have to be on a one-to-one basis. For example, if, for every increase of two units on the X axis, there is a corresponding five units decrease on the Y axis, this too would be a perfect negative relationship.

It must be recognized that a correlation of +.82 and −.82 is exactly the same size of relationship. Whether *r* is positive or negative indicates nothing more than the direction of the relationship.

Example

If the number of grams of glucose in a liter of distilled water is doubled, the osmolality of that solution is doubled. A 10% D/W solution has twice the osmolality of a 5% D/W solution. This is an example of a perfect positive relationship.

Example

Boyle's law states that at a constant temperature, the pressure of a confined gas varies inversely with the volume. Simply stated, this means that if the pressure on a gas is doubled, the volume will be exactly halved. This is an example of a perfect negative correlation.

The Pearson *r* of 0

An *r* of 0 indicates no linear regression between two variables. Linear regression is a statistic that shows how the points on a scattergram tend to cluster around a straight line. (See below.) Figure 16.4 is a scattergram which shows exam scores that have little or no such

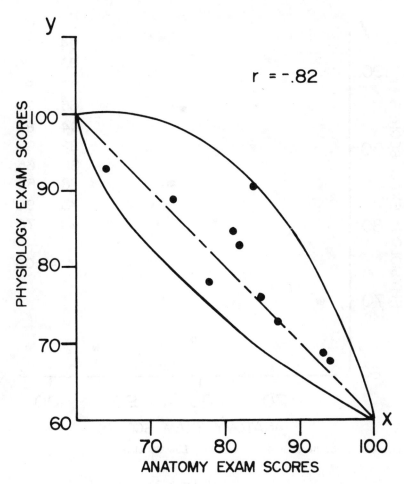

Figure 16.3. Scattergram of Data, Table 16.3

relationship. Mathematically, the Pearson *r* of scores shown in Figure 16.4 is −.06, which means nothing. An *r* of −.06 is not statistically significant. Actually, just a glance at Figure 16.4 shows that figuring the Pearson *r* would be a waste of time. (Discussion of the Pearson *r* for curvilinear regression, which may have an *r* of 0, is beyond the scope of this text.)

The Multiple Correlation Coefficient (*R*)

The multiple correlation coefficient measures the maximum relationship obtained between several independent variables (defined in next section) in order to predict a single dependent variable. For example,

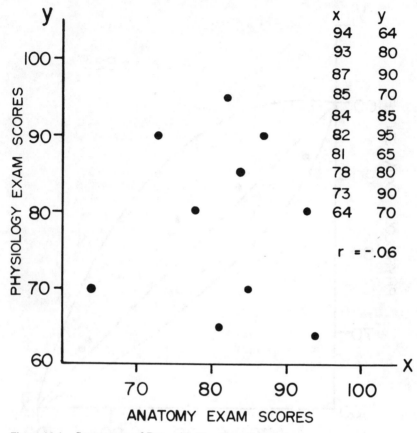

Figure 16.4. Scattergram of Data with Very Low Correlation

grade point averages in high school, scholastic aptitude test scores, and the college entrance exam scores can all be used in combination to predict success in college.

Rho, or Spearman Rank-Order Correlation Coefficient (ρ)

The Spearman rank-order correlation coefficient measures the relationship between two variables, the scores of which are all arranged in rank order; ρ is the product-moment correlation coefficient for ranked data, and can be interpreted the same as r. It is a good substitute for r when the number of cases is small. Rho is of no value when there is a large number of scores since it would be simpler to compute the Pearson r.

LINEAR REGRESSION

In order to use the Pearson *r*, scattergrams such as Figures 16.2, 16.3, and 16.4 must be analyzed to see if the points tend to fall in a straight line. This condition is known as linear regression between the two variables being studied. Linear regression describes how scores tend to cluster around a straight line.

The whole purpose of *r* is to have a means of predicting the score on one variable from the result of another variable. A common use of *r* is predicting the degree of success a student will have in college from high school grades or college entrance exams. The grade-point average made in high school is known as the predictor or the *independent variable*. The grade-point average predicted is known as the *dependent variable*. The Pearson *r*, however, cannot be used if one of the variables is controlled, which often is the case in medical experiments. When interpreting *r*, three very important points must be remembered:

1. *r* does not necessarily indicate causation.
    Example: There may be a +*r* between medical students' grade-point averages and their fathers' incomes, but their fathers' incomes are not the cause of the students' grade-point averages.
    Example: On the other hand, Boyle's law proves that with constant temperature, the volume of a gas will be halved if the pressure is doubled: the Pearson $r = -1.00$, a perfect negative correlation. In this instance, the increased pressure does cause the reduction in volume of the gas, so the perfect negative correlation does indicate that variation in one variable (gas pressure) causes a consistent variation in the other variable (gas volume).

2. *r* should not be thought of as a percentage, because, although increase in size of *r* is associated with an increase in relationship, the units of increase are often not equal, and hence cannot be interpreted as a percent.

3. *r* is greatly affected if the range of scores is narrow.
    Example: If five of the 30 medical students studied in Chap. 13 are ranked by their scores on two tests, thus:

Student	Test *A*	Test *B*
A	1	2
B	2	1
C	3	5
D	4	3
E	5	4

note that since the range is only 5, student C's change of 2 in rank equals 40%. But if he were third and fifth in rank with his 30 classmates, the change of 2 in rank would equal only 6.6%. Therefore, the Pearson r with such a narrow range of raw scores is lowered so much that it is meaningless.

STANDARD ERROR OF THE ESTIMATE

A regression equation is used to predict scores on the dependent variable. Since predictions are never 100% accurate, the amount of error involved is measured by a statistic known as the *standard error of the estimate*. If r is high between two variables, error is small, but if r is low, the error is large. The standard error of the estimate is, in reality, a standard deviation from the regression line (equation).

Suppose a National College Entrance Examination x is designed to predict college grade-point averages. This exam has a positive correlation coefficient with college grade-point averages (GPA) of .5(r = +.5), which is a reasonably good predictor. Figure 16.5 is a very rough graph of such an exam, and is designed only to demonstrate what a standard error of the estimate means. The steps below should be followed as Figure 16.5 is examined.

1. The dotted black line is the regression line and indicates the mean ($\overline{X}$) grade-point average in college that applicants with given raw scores on exam x will make. For example, applicants who make a raw score of 100 on exam x will make a mean grade point average in college of 83 (see dotted arrows on both axes).
2. The standard error of the estimate has been figured by formula for this exam to be ±4 GPA points. This is actually one standard deviation from the regression line and is represented by the two dashed black lines parallel to the regression line, which are labeled ± 4. The normal curve shows the normal distribution of college GPA for a raw score of 100. Applicants who make a raw score of 100 have a 68% chance of having their GPA fall within the band of 83 ± 4 points (79-87), as indicated by the dashed black arrows on both axes.
3. Two standard errors of the estimate (two standard deviations from the regression line) is represented by the two solid black lines parallel to the regression line. They are labeled ± 8. Applicants who make a raw score of 100 have a 95% chance of having their college grade-point averages fall within a band of 83 ± 8 points (75-91), as indicated by solid black arrows on both axes.

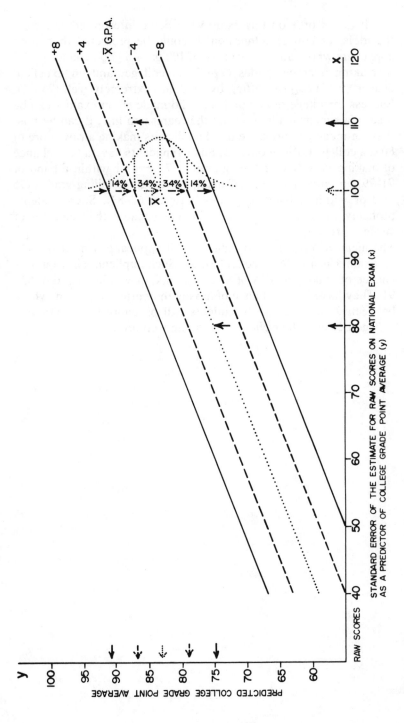

Figure 16.5.   Standard Error of the Estimate (See text)

   If raw scores on this exam were being interpreted as one of the tools for college admission, it could be predicted that those applicants who made a raw score of 100 have a good chance (68%) of making average grades (79-87) in college, and an excellent chance (95%) of just getting by or doing extremely well (75-91).

4. Success in college of an applicant who made 80 on exam x can be read in a similar manner. From the regression line, it can be read that the mean performance of all applicants making a raw score of 80 is a college GPA of only 75. Such applicants have a 68% chance of making very low or failing grades (75 ± 4 or within a band of 71-79) and a 95% chance of making average or failing grades (75 ± 8 or within a band of grades between 67-83). Such students probably will not be admitted to college because their chances of success are very poor.

5. The mean (average) performance of all applicants who make 110 on exam x is a GPA in college of 87. Such applicants have a 68% chance of making a GPA of 87 ± 4 points, or within a band of 83-91. They have a 95% chance of having their grades fall somewhere between 79 and 95. Such students will probably be admitted to college because their chances of doing well are excellent.

Chapter 17
TESTING
HYPOTHESES—
THE SIGNIFICANCE
OF DIFFERENCES

NULL HYPOTHESIS (H$_0$)

The place to start to see if apparent results from an experiment are real, or whether they are caused just by chance, is to test the experimental data with the *null hypothesis*. The null hypothesis is a statement that there is no real difference between observed results in the experimental data and in the control data. In medical research, controlled studies are generally done when the researcher wants to compare the effectiveness of a new treatment with the known effectiveness of an old or standard treatment, which then becomes his control. When he subjects his experimental data to the null hypothesis, he is testing to see if the apparent results seen in the experiment are caused by chance. The use of the null hypothesis may seem to be ambiguous or paradoxical because the researcher must assume the exact opposite of what he is trying to prove.

Level of Statistical Significance for Testing the Null Hypothesis

$p = .05$ or 5% level of significance

Much of the research data in social sciences and education is tested by the null hypothesis at the $p = .05$ level of significance. If the data meet these requirements, the null hypothesis is rejected at the $p = .05$ level. If, however, the null hypothesis proves that the observed experimental results could have been chance results in more than 5 of 100 trials, the null hypothesis is accepted as true or valid. There is, then, *no significant difference* between the mean of the control data and the mean of the experimental data. This is to say, for example, that the experimental test is, in reality, no better than the old test with which it is being compared, or that the new treatment is no better than the old traditional treatment. If the null hypothesis cannot be rejected, the experimental data are considered to be of no statistical significance. Experimentation with that particular test usually stops at that point.

$p = .01$ or 1% level of significance

Much medical research is done at the $p = .01$ level of significance. If the experimental data cannot meet the $p = .01$ level of significance, the data observed in the experiment are considered to be of no statistical significance, so the null hypothesis is valid. Since there is no *real* difference between the mean of the control and the mean of the experimental data, the difference observed in the experiment is considered to have been caused by *chance*. If, however, the data meet the $p = .01$ level of significance test, the null hypothesis is rejected at that level. The differences observed in the experiment are adequately shown to be real differences, and therefore are of statistical significance. There is only one chance in 100 that the observed results were caused by chance. If the null hypothesis can be rejected, the researcher can then make probability statements about the success of his work.

Other levels of significance

It is possible to make more stringent tests than $p = .01$. The $p = .001$ level of significance states that only one in 1,000 times could the results of an experiment be caused by chance alone. But 999 times in 1,000 a real difference between the mean of the control, and the mean of the experimental data exists. Such a level of significance is so stringent that research data must be extremely good to meet this criterion.

TESTING SIGNIFICANCE OF DIFFERENCES

In making tests of significance, z scores are generally used. Standard z scores were studied in Chap. 16. Recall that $\pm 3z$ has the same numerical value as ± 3 standard deviations (see Fig. 16.1). If the percentages of scores that lie under the normal curve are added, $\pm 2s$ includes 95.44% of the scores (See Fig. 14.6): $\pm 3s$ includes 99.74% of the scores. Since a z score has the same numerical value as a standard deviation:

z scores lying between $\pm 2z$ include 95.44% of the scores
z scores lying between $\pm 3z$ include 99.74% of the scores

The objective of calculating the z score for experimental data is to see how large a z score it can make—the larger the z score, the more statistically significant the experimental results. If the z score is large enough, the null hypothesis can be rejected. If the null hypothesis can be rejected, the researcher can then make probability statements about the success of his experiment. However, if the z score is too small, the null hypothesis of no difference between the experimental and the control data must be accepted as valid because the small z score proves that there is too much of an element of chance playing a significant or real part in the observed results of the experiment. When the null hypothesis must be accepted as valid, the experiment is probably worthless. (There are, however, some situations when the researcher wants to demonstrate that there is no difference between the experimental and the control data, and is trying to show that the null hypothesis is valid (see examples, Chap. 19).

Tables of z scores in statistical texts show that z scores lying between ± 1.96 include exactly 95% of the scores, and z scores of ± 2.58 include exactly 99% of the scores. If a z score lies between ± 1.96 and ± 2.58, the null hypothesis can be rejected at the $p = .05$ level of significance. Such a statistic can be written: $p < .05$, or $p \le .05$, or $.05 > p > .01$. Any one of these statistics means that the probability of chance is less than 5%.

If the z score is larger than ± 2.58, the null hypothesis can be rejected at the $p = .01$ level of significance. Sometimes such a level of significance is written: $p < .01$ or $p \le .01$ or $.01 > p > .001$ (see Chap. 15, *Confidence Levels and Intervals*).

Steps in Testing Significance of Data

1. The researcher states the null hypothesis of no difference between results of his experiment and the control data.
2. He predetermines the level of statistical significance at which he will reject the null hypothesis. If the researcher elects to risk $p = .05$ level of significance, he must ask, "Is the result of my experiment 1 of the 5 in 100 that are caused by chance?" Maybe it is! That is the risk he is willing to take. In medical experiments, researchers must be extremely cautious in making predictions because human lives are often the gamble. Requiring p to equal .01 is the rigorous test of the null hypothesis that medical experimentation generally demands. The element of chance playing a part in experimental results must always be considered and shown by statistical tests to be extremely low before the results can be accepted by the medical profession, even for experimental use on human beings.
3. He figures the z score for his data.
4. The z score will tell him at what level of significance he can reject the null hypothesis. (If he elected to reject it at $p = .01$, he can

do so, providing his z score is 2.58 or more. If his z score is less than 2.58, the null hypothesis is considered to be valid.)

Testing the Significance of Differences Between Means

One of the most common ways that medical research is done is by controlled trial. The controlled trial is a method used to compare the effectiveness of a new drug or treatment with that of an old, standard drug or treatment. Often it is very difficult to find two or more groups of patients or animals so much alike that no outside factor or circumstance can have any bearing on the outcome of the study. With this in mind, the hypothetical data below are used to demonstrate the test of significance of differences between means.

An experiment is being done with a new drug A as a cure for disease D. Researchers wish to compare the data compiled by use of new drug A with data available for traditional drug B, the control. Below are the cure rate statistics for the two drugs:

New Drug A	Traditional Drug B (control)
$\bar{X} = 62$	$\bar{X} = 59$
$N_A = 100$ patients	$N_B = 150$ patients
$s_A = 7.5$	$s_B = 6.4$

Step 1   The null hypothesis of no *real* difference between the means of the two groups is stated. The null hypothesis asserts that there is no *real* difference between the effectiveness of the two drugs A and B in curing disease D. It compares the mean of A with the mean of B, stating that they both come from the same population (all patients cured with traditional drug B), and any observed difference in cure rates is caused by chance.

Subtract the mean of B from the mean of A.

$62 - 59 = 3$

H_0 states that $\bar{X}_A - \bar{X}_B = 0$.

The null hypothesis assumes that the actual difference of 3 is a *chance* deviation from a mean difference of 0. It is believed by the researcher that this chance deviation of 3 (taking into consideration the fewer number of patients in the group testing drug A, and its standard deviation) is too large to be caused by chance alone.

Step 2   The researcher elects to submit his data to the null hypothesis at the $p = .01$ level of significance to see if he can reject it.

Step 3   From a formula appropriate for this type of data, it is calculated that $z = 3.26$.

Step 4   Since z is more than 2.58, the researcher can reject the null hypothesis at the $p < .01$ level of significance.

It should be noted that such results are a researcher's dream—z is much larger than 2.58, and the null hypothesis could be rejected at an even more stringent level than $p = .001$. The researcher has very promising results from his experiment, so he can make some very positive statements about the new drug A and its ability to cure disease D. However, if possible, he should repeat his experiment before reporting it. When interpreting data of this type in professional reading, the number of persons, or instances, in the experiment is extremely important. The more there are in both groups, the more reliable the data will be. If the study has been repeated by other investigators with essentially the same results, the report is all the more reliable. Thus it is well to pay attention to any references to other studies submitted with the report.

Other Examples of z Scores

If the z score $= 1.79$, the null hypothesis is valid, and the experiment is statistically insignificant. Tables of z scores indicate that a z score of 1.79 is equivalent to $p = .073$, which means that there is more than a 7% chance that the differences observed between the two groups studied occurred by chance.

If the z score equals 2.37, the null hypothesis can be rejected at $p < .05$.

If the z score equals 2.59, the null hypothesis can be rejected at $p < .01$.

If the z score equals 1.95, the null hypothesis is valid. The experiment is statistically insignificant. A z score must be at *least* ± 1.96 to be statistically significant at the $p = .05$ level of significance.

Testing the Significance of Differences Between Proportions

The test of significance for differences between proportions and percentages is done statistically by a specific formula with much the same rationale as for testing the significance of differences between means:

Step 1   The null hypothesis of no *real* difference between the proportions is stated.

Step 2   The researcher predetermines the level of significance at which he wishes to reject the null hypothesis (usually $p = .05$, or $p = .01$).

Step 3   From a formula appropriate for this type of data, the z score is calculated.

Step 4   The null hypothesis is accepted as valid or rejected as dictated by the z score.

Since proportions and percentages are so similar, percentages are determined simply by multiplying the proportion by 100.

The *chi-square* test of significance can also be used to figure the significance of differences between proportions. See below.

Testing the Significance of Differences Between Medians

Testing the difference between sampling distributions of medians is also done by specific formula in much the same manner as testing the differences between means and proportions:

Step 1   The null hypothesis of no *real* difference between the medians is stated.

Step 2   The researcher predetermines the level of significance at which he wishes to reject the null hypothesis.

Step 3   From a formula appropriate for this type of data, the z score is calculated.

Step 4   The null hypothesis is accepted as valid, or rejected, as dictated by the z score.

Testing the Significance of the Pearson r (Product-Moment Correlation Coefficient)

When the Pearson r is used in medical experimentation, it is always checked by the null hypothesis for a high level of significance (at least $p = .01$) before using it in further computations. From Table 16.2, it was calculated that $r = +.84$ between the scores made in anatomy and physiology exams given to 10 medical students. Is this r of $+.84$ valid? Are the two exams *really* correlated, or does this apparently very high r occur as a chance deviation from the population R of 30 medical students? The null hypothesis states that there is no real relationship between the scores made on the two exams by the entire class of 30 medical students. However, the sample of 10 medical students out of a class of 30 is a very large sample, so $r = +.84$ should be very significant. Nevertheless, if the grades of these 10 students had been used to predict the relationship of anatomy exam x to physiology exam y results for all the thousands of medical students in the country, the element of chance would be so high that the null hypothesis of no relationship between the two exams would be valid, and the r obtained would be statistically insignificant. The smaller the size of a sample in relation to the population, the greater the possibility that chance enters into the computations.

Testing the significance of the Pearson r

Step 1   The null hypothesis is stated. It asserts that the population $R = 0$. In the example given above, this statement means that the

r of +.84 obtained between the scores made on the anatomy and physiology exams taken by the 10 medical students is just a chance deviation from the population R, which is really 0. In other words, the null hypothesis states that there is no real relationship between the grades made on the anatomy exam and those made on the physiology exam. The apparent relationship between the grades made by the 10 medical students is a result caused entirely by chance.

Step 2   The desired level of significance is predetermined.

Step 3   A statistical table shows that, in this particular situation, if r = .84, the null hypothesis can be rejected at p = .01 level of significance.

TESTING SIGNIFICANCE WITH CHI-SQUARE (χ^2)

When a new and very useful test of significance was first computed, statisticians elected to designate it by the 22nd letter of the Greek alphabet χ, known as "chi" (pronounced kī), and written χ^2. Care should be taken not to confuse χ^2 with the commonly used English letter X and X^2.

Later in this discussion it will be seen that the value for *chi-square* is closely related to z^2. How the statistic z is used as a test of significance has already been discussed. The discussion about tests of significance up to this point has concerned statistics involved with assumed normal distributions in the population, and with tests that can measure only one difference at a time.

The use of chi-square as a test of significance permits the testing of several differences at the same time and makes no assumption that the population distribution is normal. Chi-square can also be used as a substitute for problems testing differences between proportions, as was mentioned before. The chi-square equation can be used as a test of the null hypothesis of no significant difference between two or more groups.

The general formula for chi-square is:

$$\chi^2 = \text{the sum of } \frac{(\text{observed frequencies} - \text{expected frequencies})^2}{\text{expected frequencies}}$$

For the simplest possible example, suppose a penny is tossed 20 times, and it comes up heads 15 times and tails 5 times. It would be expected that it would come up heads 10 times and tails 10 times. Does the above result mean that the penny is not balanced or is "fixed?" Submitting the data to the chi-square equation can answer this question:

$$\chi^2 = \frac{(\text{observed heads} - \text{expected heads})^2}{\text{expected heads}}$$

$$+ \frac{(\text{observed tails} - \text{expected tails})^2}{\text{expected tails}}$$

$$\chi^2 = \frac{(15 - 10)^2}{10} + \frac{(5 - 10)^2}{10}$$

$$= \frac{(5)^2}{10} + \frac{(-5)^2}{10} = 25/10 + 25/10$$

$$\chi^2 = 2.5 + 2.5 = 5$$

The chi-square table in a statistical textbook indicates that, in this specific situation, when χ^2 is 5, the null hypothesis can be rejected at the $p < .05$ level of significance. The penny, therefore, probably is not balanced. It has been shown statistically that if 100 perfectly balanced pennies are individually tossed 20 times, only 5 of the 100 pennies will come up heads 15 times. Is this penny one of these 5? It might be. If the researcher rejects the null hypothesis at the $p = .05$ level of significance, that is the chance he is willing to take. This use of the chi-square formula checks to see whether observed data is really different from expected data. In this example, the researcher is gambling that his penny is not one of the five that are expected to come up heads 15 times, and that his penny is really different from the 100 perfectly balanced pennies.

From this illustration, it can be seen that, if the observed frequencies are very close to the expected frequencies, chi-square will be small, but if there is a large difference between the observed and the expected frequencies, chi-square will be large. Therefore, small values for chi-square point to the validity of the null hypothesis, and large values for chi-square will lead to its rejection.

Uses of Chi-Square

Chi-square has a great many uses in statistics. Whenever the expected frequencies for a normal distribution can be figured by formula for a set of observed data, the chi-square formula can be used as a test of significance. The null hypothesis states that the observed distribution is a chance variation from a normal distribution. If the null hypothesis can be rejected at the $p = .01$ level of significance, it means that the observed differences are so great that only one time in 100 would a sampling so different from the normal curve occur by chance alone. Such a test of the null hypothesis is known as the chi-square test of *goodness of fit*, or how the observed data "fit" into the population normal distribution (see Chap. 19, problem 8).

The chi-square formula is the same for all research situations. The difference in its use is related to differences in research methods used to get the observed and expected frequencies, and then in its interpretation.

Relationship of χ^2 to z^2

A discussion of degrees of freedom is beyond the scope of this text. It is enough to know that they relate to sample size. But it is interesting to note that when there is one degree of freedom in interpretation:

$$\chi^2 = z^2$$

When $p = .05$, z score $= \pm1.96$. (See above, *Testing Significance of Differences*.)

$$z^2 = (\pm1.96)^2 = 3.841$$

With 1 degree of freedom:

$$\text{When } p = .05, \chi^2 = 3.841$$

$$\sqrt{3.841} = \pm1.96$$

SUMMARY

When the null hypothesis can be rejected at $p = .01$, the researcher has reason to believe that his research data are significantly different from the control data. Then he must ask himself how they are different. Only the first milestone has been passed in the testing process, and each step of the way the accumulated data must be subjected to at least one of the tests of significance.

There are a great many tests of significance. Chi-square is just one of them that is particularly useful because it has such versatility. All the tests are designed to test the null hypothesis of no difference between experimental and control data. Results of the test of the null hypothesis are generally interpreted by use of a statistical table designed for use with the specific test. The predetermined level of significance can be read directly from the table and the null hypothesis is accepted as valid or rejected accordingly. Since the sole purpose of this discussion is to learn to interpret statistical symbols encountered in the professional literature, it is only necessary to understand that all these tests of significance merely state what statistical test was used, and at what level of significance the null hypothesis was rejected. The reader must then use his own judgment in accepting the claims made. He should search for other studies that substantiate claims made by any article he reads. He should ask:

1. Is the level of significance at which the researcher rejected the null hypothesis adequate for the particular study in question? Is the element of chance playing too large a part in the results?
2. Was the study repeated at least once, or are there other articles that support the results of this study?
3. Is the number of persons or items in the samples tested in the study large enough in relation to the population to make the claims valid?
4. Are the controls adequate?
5. Is the study biased in any way? If so, how?

It must be mentioned that controlled studies are quite difficult to set up. It is often very hard to find two groups that are so much alike that no outside factor or circumstance can have any bearing on the outcome of the study. For this reason, biased experiments are the rule rather than the exception. The critical reader must always look for bias when assessing the controls used in any experiment.

If, for example, the researcher uses all young and healthy persons or animals rather than a true random sample for his experiment, and then compares the results of his experiment with the traditional method used on true random samples, the study is biased.

Sometimes researchers are tempted to drop subjects that deviate radically from the desired results of the experiment. Sometimes when a new drug is tested, one or more patients are forced to drop out of the study due to serious toxic side effects. However, such subjects should not be excluded from the study. If they are not included in the final report, the results of the study are likely to be extremely biased. Perhaps the use of the new drug may be seriously compromised by its tendency to cause toxic side effects.

The same study done by two researchers is rarely identical unless elaborate guidelines are set up and followed meticulously by both researchers.

The same study done at two different laboratories will differ considerably, because procedures for testing are different. This is the reason many hospital laboratories have different norms for their various tests.

Double-blind studies have been used as a common method to avoid bias. By use of this method, neither the researcher nor the patient knows which of two (or more) drugs or treatments is being used.

There are many tests of significance not mentioned in this text.

Their uses are predominantly in the social sciences, education, business, etc. and they are used only occasionally by researchers in the medical sciences. If they are encountered in the medical literature, their meaning should be evident from the text that describes the experiment. They will all involve some statistical method for determining whether the data presented are statistically significant at a predetermined level of significance. The data will always be subjected to at least one of the tests of the null hypothesis of no difference between the results of the experiment, and the control data.

It must be emphasized that professional literature is loaded with experiments that cannot be duplicated. A researcher in the medical sciences should try to repeat his experiment, if possible, before reporting it. The reason for this recommendation is that, regardless of the level at which a researcher rejects the null hypothesis, he should prove to himself that he has not made any gross miscalculations in his data. In addition, repeating the study will help to prove that the result of his research is not one of those due to chance.

Chapter 18
RELIABILITY
AND VALIDITY

RELIABILITY

Reliability Calculated from the Pearson *r*

Reliability means consistency. One of the chief uses of correlation coefficients is to measure the consistency with which an examination or experiment performs. Can the exam in question be relied upon to give the same results every time it is given to the same person? Rarely is the same exam or medical test given repeatedly to the same person. Therefore, at least two comparable (called "parallel") tests are given to each person and the results of the two tests are then correlated to see how closely they relate to each other. The Pearson *r* in this case is interpreted as being the *reliability* of the test.

Sometimes reliability is tested by computing two scores on a long examination. Odd numbered questions are scored and totaled, and then even numbered questions are scored and totaled. The two totals are submitted to the Pearson *r* equation, and the result obtained is the reliability of the examination.

Errors in the reliability of a test may be the result of daily differences in the health or emotions of an individual who takes the test, guessing, incorrect interpretation of a question, etc. Factors such as these cause the error component of the test, and the higher the error component, the lower the *r* of the reliability of the test will be. Generally speaking, the longer the test (within fatigue limits), the more reliable it will be.

Thus, the reliability coefficient should be high: *r* should equal .8 or more, as a rule. However, it is a relative measurement, and the situation surrounding the use of the statistic should be taken into account.

Reliability Determined from the Standard Error of the Measurement

Another method for determining the reliability of a test or experiment is to figure the *standard error of the measurement*. For example, suppose a sample of blood was drawn from a healthy individual, hourly, for 10 successive hours and a hypothetical test for mg of abc/L of blood was performed on each sample. The results obtained would be very close to the same but not identical. If the mean of the reports calculated from the 10 samples was figured, it could be used as an estimate of this individual's true value for abc/L of blood. The standard deviation of the 10 sample values from this individual's true (mean) value is known as the standard error of the measurement.

Such repetition of a test to the same person is unrealistic, so the standard error of the measurement is estimated by a statistical formula. The reliability of every laboratory test, which allows for variation in the way the technician performs the test, reads the results, etc., is judged by this estimated standard error of the measurement. The individual's "true value" lies within a band of ± the standard error of the measurement from the raw measurement of one test performed by the technician. Therefore, since the standard error of the measurement is, in reality, a standard deviation, a patient's true value for a particular lab test can be 99% relied upon to lie within a band of ± 3 standard errors of the measurement from the raw numerical value that appears on his lab report. As might be expected, the smaller the standard error of the measurement, the more reliable the test is. All laboratory reports should be interpreted with the standard error of the measurement in mind.

VALIDITY

Chapter 16 discussed the fact that predictions are never 100% accurate, and that a statistic known as the standard error of the estimate can measure the amount of error involved in making predictions. As an example of the use of this statistic, raw scores made on a college entrance examination were discussed as a method for predicting success in college.

Did this particular college entrance exam really test what it was alleged to test? Just how accurate, for example, are the grades made on this particular college entrance exam in predicting success in college? *Predictive validity* statistics answer these questions.

For example: To validate this particular college entrance examination, a group of college applicants was given this examination, and after they had completed their freshman year, their grade-point averages and the grades they made on the college entrance exam were correlated by use of the Pearson *r* equation. The validity *r* thus reached is the validity of this particular college entrance exam as a predictor of success in college.

Validity correlation coefficients are, for the most part, much lower than reliability *r*, and fall within the range of .4–.6. The reason for this low validity r is that no test can predict motivation, health of the student when he takes the examination versus his health while a student in college, or distractions such as outside employment, emotional attachments, use of drugs, etc. No doubt everyone has known students who have had very high grade-point averages in high school, but did not do well in college. Everyone has also known some students who made low grades in high school, but suddenly "got with it", and did extremely well in college. For these reasons, $r = .5$ is considered to be a reasonably good validity correlation for an exam used as a predictor of success. Obviously, the higher the validity correlation, the better is the prediction for the dependent variable.

POST SCRIPT

As was pointed out above, the objective is solely to help the student interpret the statistics he constantly encounters in his professional reading. Admittedly, the discussion is oversimplified in an effort to make the material not only simple, but also easily understandable and brief. Undoubtedly there are a great many questions that are not answered in this discussion. If the student needs a more extensive explanation of any part of statistical analysis, he is urged to study any of the excellent statistical textbooks available. Statistics should not intimidate him—compiling statistics is more tedious than it is difficult.

Chapter 19
PROBLEMS INVOLVING INTERPRETATION OF STATISTICAL SYMBOLS

The following statistical results might be found supporting statements in a professional journal. A brief discussion of each problem appears at the end of this chapter.

Problems 1-6 concern various hypothetical statistics concerned with a new drug xyz, and its effect on serum abc.

1. Mean serum abc level was 13.2 mg/ml for 268 subjects taking experimental drug xyz, as compared with 13.7 mg/ml for 236 control subjects taking no drug. The difference between these values is not significant ($p > .1$).
   Why is ($p > .1$) not significant?
   When could a result such as this be desired by the researcher?

2. There was a significant correlation between test d and test f for serum abc values ($r = .44$, $p < .01$).
   What does $r = .44$ indicate?
   What does $p < .01$ mean as far as the Pearson r is concerned in this example?

3. The mean hemoglobin level of the 268 subjects taking the drug xyz, was 12.4 g/100 ml, as compared with 11.8 g/100 ml for the 236 control subjects. The difference between these values is statistically significant ($p < .001$).
   Why is this report statistically significant?

4. There was no significant difference in the mean red blood cell volume between the two groups ($p > .05$).
   Why is this statement not significant?
   How could this result possibly be desired by the researcher?

5.   An earlier study in this laboratory with smaller sample numbers analyzed immediately after collection of the specimen showed a strong correlation ($r = .83$) between test d and test f level for serum abc. The lower correlation ($r = .44$) obtained in the present study probably reflects the expected variations in sampling, processing, storing, and testing of large numbers of samples inherent in this study.

Should this explanation of the lower correlation in the present study be accepted as valid?

6.   The hemoglobin level (mean $\pm$ $s_{\bar{x}}$) for the group being treated with drug xyz was 12.4 g/100 ml $\pm$ .2 g ($p < .01$). The hemoglobin level for the control group taking no drug was 11.8 g/100 ml $\pm$ .3 g ($p \leq .01$).

Explain the significance of the standard error of the mean in this example.

7.   The disease incidence among children less than 5 years of age living in a low-income, high-density neighborhood (105/100,000/annum) was significantly higher ($p < .0005$) than that among children less than 5 years of age living in a middle-class neighborhood (76/100,000/annum).

Exactly what does "$p < .0005$" mean in this statement?

8.   The distribution of the incidence of this disease in the 105 patients observed is grouped according to median family income in Figure 19.1. The upper histogram shows the number of cases expected in each category of income on the basis of disease incidence recorded by the Department of Health in this state. The lower histogram shows the observed number of cases.

Explain the chi-square "goodness of fit" test of the null hypothesis as it is used in the accompanying histograms.

9.   Under a chart that contains chi-square analysis of the effectiveness of a drug in killing different strains of bacteria is the following statement:

"Significance was defined as $\chi^2 > 3.9$ ($p \leq .05$)."

Exactly what does this statement mean?

10. The reliability of a specific laboratory test is judged by the calculated standard error of the measurement. Why should one laboratory report be judged with the calculated standard error of the measurement in mind? What is the patient's true value?

DISCUSSION OF PROBLEMS

1.   "$p > .1$" means that the probability of the results occurring by chance is greater than 10 in 100 samples. In this instance, the

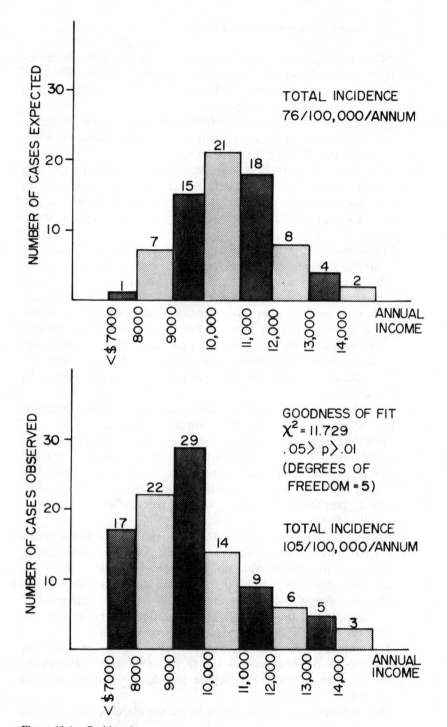

Figure 19.1. Problem 8

217

difference in the mean serum abc level in the 268 subjects taking the experimental drug xyz is considered to be a chance difference from the mean serum abc level of the 236 subjects in the control group taking no drug.

Such a result could be desired by the researcher if he wanted to demonstrate that the experimental drug xyz does not have any significant effect on the serum abc level.

2. When r is .44 there is a positive correlation between the two tests for serum abc. Such a correlation indicates that the statistics accumulated by the use of these two tests tend to be associated, i.e.: test d produces similar results to those of test f for serum abc.

    In this example, $p < .01$ is the null hypothesis test of significance for the Pearson r. The null hypothesis states that the r of .44 obtained between test d and test f for serum abc is just a chance deviation from the population R, which is really 0, i.e.: there is no real relationship between the two tests, and the apparent relationship between them is a result caused entirely by chance. The $p < .01$ level of significance indicates the point where the null hypothesis was rejected. Only one time in 100 would such a correlation between the two tests be caused by chance.

3. ''$p < .001$'' is significant because it indicates that only one time in 1,000 could such a result be caused by chance.

4. This statement is not significant because the results in the study could have been caused by chance in more than five in 100 tests.

    The researcher might have wanted the two groups to have identical mean red blood volumes, thereby eliminating the possibility that the new drug xyz had an adverse effect on red blood cell volume.

5. A second study showed that the two tests, d and f, for serum abc had less of a correlation (or similarity) than an earlier study. However, the studies were not the same:
    a) The number of samples in the second study was much larger.
    b) The serum samples were stored (frozen? refrigerated? dried?) and processed later in a different way. In the first study, the samples were analyzed immediately.

    The researcher justifies the lower correlation as being caused by expected variations such as the factors mentioned. The explanation given should be accepted guardedly. Further study is needed.

6. The standard error of the mean is the standard deviation of the

means of a sampling distribution. The statement

$$\overline{X} \pm s_{\overline{x}} = 12.4 \text{ g/100 ml} \pm .2 \text{ g } (p < .01)$$

assures the reader that there is a 99+% certainty that the mean hemoglobin level of the population taking drug xyz will fall within the range of 12.2–12.6 g/100 ml. The statement

$$\overline{X} \pm s_{\overline{x}} = 11.8 \text{ g/100 ml} \pm .3 \text{ g/100 ml } (p \leq .01)$$

indicates that there is less than one chance in 100 that the mean hemoglobin level of the population taking no drug will fall outside the range of 11.5–12.1 g/100 ml.

7. "$p < .0005$" means that in less than 5 in 10,000 (1 in 2,000) such studies would such a large difference between the disease incidence in the two groups be caused by chance. The implication is that the disease incidence among poor children less than 5 years of age was much higher than among middle-class children of the same age. (This statement, taken out of context, should not be accepted *per se*. The discussion in the article about the study must substantiate such a claim.)

8. The chi-square "goodness of fit" test of the null hypothesis states that the median family income in the group studied has no more or less effect on the incidence of this disease than the median family income has on the incidence of the disease throughout the entire state. The chi-square equation assumes that any difference between the lower histogram (the group studied) and the upper histogram (a normal distribution of the disease incidence throughout the state) is caused by chance.

    The null hypothesis is rejected at $.05 > p > .01$. This statistic means that a difference from the control in the incidence of this disease, as was observed in this one sample, could have occurred by chance in less than 5 in 100 samples, but in more than 1 in 100 samples. The null hypothesis is rejected at the $p = .05$ level of significance. The observed sample does not fit into the normal distribution of the control. (A close look at the two histograms shows that 17 of the 105 cases observed reported annual family incomes of less than $7,000. This is a large deviation from the incidence of only one case per 100,000 population expected in children whose families have an annual income of less than $7,000.)

9. The chi-square table in a statistical textbook indicates that if $\chi^2 = 3.841$, $p = .05$. Therefore, if $\chi^2 > 3.9$, p will be less than .05.

(The larger the value of chi-square, the lower is the possibility that the results of the study were caused by chance.) Only 5 times in 100 trials could the bacteria have been killed by factors other than those indicated in the chart.

10. The standard error of the measurement allows for such variations as the way the technician performs the test or reads results. The patient's "true" value lies within a band of ± the standard error of the measurement from the raw value of the one laboratory report. This raw measurement can be 99% relied upon to fall within ± 3 standard errors of the measurement for that particular test.

APPENDIX

A BRIEF REVIEW OF FRACTIONS AND DECIMALS

This appendix is designed for the student who has difficulty working with fractions and decimals. Weakness in this type of mathematics is very common, and probably is not the fault of the student, but may well be due to the method by which he was taught mathematics in grade school.

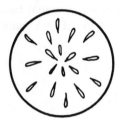

The circle on the left represents 1 whole pie.

Usually 1 whole pie is cut, before serving, into parts or fractions of the whole pie.

FRACTIONS

A fraction is a part of a whole. If 1 whole pie is cut into 4 equal parts, there still would be 1 pie, but it now is in 4 equal pieces, with each part equal to one-fourth of the whole pie. This fact is expressed as 1/4, which technically is known as a fraction.

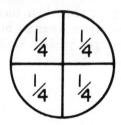

$$\frac{1}{4} + \frac{1}{4} + \frac{1}{4} + \frac{1}{4} = \frac{4}{4} = 1 \text{ whole pie}$$

If 1 of the 4 equal pieces of pie has been eaten, by subtraction it can be calculated that 3/4 of the pie is left:

$$\frac{4}{4} - \frac{1}{4} = \frac{3}{4}$$

The numbers in a fraction are the terms of the fraction. The terms of the fraction 3/4 are labeled thus:

3 is the numerator (dividend). It indicates the number of parts of the whole pie that are left.

4 is the denominator (divisor). It indicates the number of parts that make up the whole pie, or the number of parts into which the whole pie is divided.

The line between the 3 and the 4 means divided by.

Therefore, the fraction 3/4 literally means 3 ÷ 4, or 3 of 4 equal parts. If the numerator is smaller than the denominator, the fraction is known as a *common* or *proper fraction* because it represents less than 1 whole unit, in this case, 1 whole pie.

If there are 2 whole pies, and each one is cut into 4 equal parts, there will be 8 equal parts, each part being 1/4 of 1 pie. This situation can be expressed by the fraction 8/4.

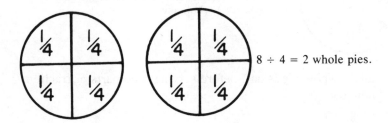

$8 \div 4 = 2$ whole pies.

If 1 of the 1/4 pieces of pie is eaten:

$$8/4 - 1/4 = 7/4 \text{ of the 2 pies are left.}$$

Since 7/4 is more than 1 whole pie, it is known as an *improper fraction.* Generally, 7/4 would be divided into a *mixed number,* and expressed as 1¾ pies left.

It is easiest to work with fractions when they are reduced to their lowest terms. A fraction is reduced to its lowest terms when its numerator and denominator cannot be divided exactly by any whole number.

Examples:

$$\frac{14 \, (\div 2) = 7}{16 \, (\div 2) = 8} \text{ reduced fraction}$$

$$\frac{6 \, (\div 3) = 2}{9 \, (\div 3) = 3} \text{ reduced fraction}$$

$$\frac{14\ (\div\ 2)\ =\ 7}{8\ (\div\ 2)\ =\ 4} = 1\ \frac{3}{4}\ \text{reduced to a mixed number}$$

(improper fraction)

Do the answers make *sense*?

Equivalent Fractions

If both the numerator and the denominator of a fraction are multiplied or divided by the same number, an equivalent fraction has been produced. In other words, both fractions have the same value.

Examples:

$$\frac{2\ (\times\ 2)\ =\ 4}{3\ (\times\ 2)\ =\ 6}$$

$$\frac{2\ (\times\ 4)\ =\ \ \ 8}{3\ (\times\ 4)\ =\ 12}$$

$$\frac{4\ (\div\ 2)\ =\ 2}{6\ (\div\ 2)\ =\ 3}$$

$$\frac{8\ (\div\ 4)\ =\ 2}{12\ (\div\ 4)\ =\ 3}$$

The student should be able to see that these answers make *sense*.

ADDITION AND SUBTRACTION OF FRACTIONS

Least (Smallest) Common (Same) Denominator (Name)

The word "denominate" means "to name". Literally, the "smallest same name" is given to fractions when they are reduced to their "least common denominator". As it is not possible to add 4 apples, 2 bananas, and 3 oranges directly as such, they are called by their "common name", which is "fruit". There are 9 pieces of fruit. Similarly, a common name, or common denominator must be found for fractions which are to be added or subtracted. To find this *common denominator*, the smallest possible number that is exactly divisible by all the denominators, and results in a whole number, is found. Then all the fractions must be changed to this common denominator.

Example 1: Addition of Fractions

$$\frac{1}{3} + \frac{1}{2}$$

The smallest possible number divisible by both 3 and 2 is 6. Therefore, 6 is the least common denominator of 3 and 2. The fractions 1/3 and 1/2 are both changed to this common denominator:

$$\text{Since } 3 \times 2 = 6 \qquad \frac{1 \times 2 = 2}{3 \times 2 = 6}$$

$$\text{Since } 2 \times 3 = 6 \qquad \frac{1 \times 3 = 3}{2 \times 3 = 6}$$

Now all that remains to be done is to add the numerators, which are the numbers or parts, as "pieces of fruit" above.

$$\frac{2}{6} + \frac{3}{6} = \frac{5}{6}$$

Example 2: Subtraction of Fractions

$$\frac{1}{2} - \frac{1}{3}$$

Again, these fractions are changed to their smallest or least common denominator. The smaller numerator is then subtracted from the larger.

$$1/2 = 3/6$$

$$1/3 = 2/6$$

$$\frac{3}{6} - \frac{2}{6} = \frac{1}{6}$$

Example 3

Add: 7/8 + 5/16 + 1/2

The least common denominator is 16, since 16 can be divided by both 8 and 2. Change 7/8 and 1/2 to 16ths.

$$7/8 = 14/16$$

$$1/2 = 8/16$$

$$\frac{14}{16} + \frac{5}{16} + \frac{8}{16} = \frac{27}{16} = 1\frac{11}{16} \text{(mixed number)}$$

Example 4

Subtract 5/16 from 1 3/16

$$1\frac{3}{16} = \frac{16}{16} + \frac{3}{16} = \frac{19}{16}$$

$$\frac{19}{16} - \frac{5}{16} = \frac{14}{16} = \frac{7}{8}$$

Since the denominators are the same, the smaller numerator is subtracted from the larger, and the resulting fraction is reduced to its lowest terms.

Example 5

Subtract 1/2 from 4/5. The least common denominator is 10.

$$4/5 = 8/10$$

$$1/2 = 5/10$$

$$8/10 - 5/10 = 3/10$$

Do these answers make *sense*?

It is important to know the relative size of various fractions, and to do this, the fractions involved must be changed to their least common denominator.

Example 6

List the following fractions in order of size from smallest to largest.

$$1/2 \quad 2/9 \quad 1/3 \quad 1/6$$

The least common denominator that is divisible by 2, 9, 3, and 6 is 18. Each fraction is changed to 18ths.

$$1/2 = 9/18 \quad 2/9 = 4/18 \quad 1/3 = 6/18 \quad 1/6 = 3/18$$

It is easy to list these fractions according to the sizes of their numerators:

$$3/18 \quad 4/18 \quad 6/18 \quad 9/18$$

They now can be reduced to the original fractions and placed in order of their relative sizes from smallest to largest:

$$1/6 \quad 2/9 \quad 1/3 \quad 1/2$$

Do the answers make *sense*?

MULTIPLICATION OF FRACTIONS

To multiply one fraction by another fraction, one numerator is multiplied by the other numerator, and one denominator is multiplied by the other denominator. Then the answer is reduced to its lowest terms:

Example 1: Multiply 1/2 × 2/3.

$$\frac{1 \times 2}{2 \times 3} = \frac{2}{6}$$

$$\text{reduced} = \frac{1}{3}$$

Example 2: Multiply 1 3/4 × 2 1/2.

First, these mixed numers must be changed to improper fractions:

$$1\frac{3}{4} = \frac{7}{4} \qquad 2\frac{1}{2} = \frac{5}{2}$$

The problem now reads:

$$\frac{7}{4} \times \frac{5}{2} = \frac{35}{8} = 4\frac{3}{8}$$

Example 3

To multiply a whole number by a fraction, treat the whole number as if it were a numerator of a fraction with a denominator of 1. Multiply 8 × 2/3.

$$\frac{8}{1} \times \frac{2}{3} = \frac{16}{3} = 5\frac{1}{3}$$

$$\text{Multiply} \quad 2 \times \frac{3}{8} = \frac{6}{8} = \frac{3}{4}$$

Reduction

To divide one of the numerators and one of the denominators by the same number is called reduction, or simplification. Sometimes it is called cancellation, but this is a misleading term because it implies that nothing is left.

Example: Multiply 3/5 × 15/18

Notice that the numerator of the first fraction, 3, and the denominator of the second fraction, 18, can both be divided by 3.

$$3 \div 3 = 1 \qquad 18 \div 3 = 6$$

Similarly, the numerator of the second fraction, 15, and the denominator of the first fraction, 5, can both be divided by 5.

$$15 \div 5 = 3 \qquad 5 \div 5 = 1$$

Generally such reduction of fractions is indicated in the following manner:

$$\frac{\overset{1}{\cancel{3}}}{\underset{1}{\cancel{5}}} \times \frac{\overset{3}{\cancel{15}}}{\underset{6}{\cancel{18}}} = \frac{3}{6} = \frac{1}{2}$$

When reduction of fractions is done in this manner, it not only makes the math simpler, but often also eliminates or simplifies the need for reducing the answer to its lowest terms. The above problem, done without reduction, would be more difficult:

$$\frac{3}{5} \times \frac{15}{18} = \frac{45}{90} = \frac{1}{2}$$

RECIPROCALS

Any whole number can be expressed as a fraction by giving it a denominator of 1.

Examples

$$4 = \frac{4}{1} \qquad 2 = \frac{2}{1} \qquad 99 = \frac{99}{1}$$

A *reciprocal* is a quantity that is inverted, or turned over:

Examples

The reciprocal of $\frac{2}{1}$ is $\frac{1}{2}$

The reciprocal of $\frac{4}{1}$ is $\frac{1}{4}$

The reciprocal of $\frac{56}{71}$ is $\frac{71}{56}$

The product of any number and its reciprocal is 1:

Example

$$\frac{2}{1} \times \frac{1}{2} = 1 \qquad \frac{4}{1} \times \frac{1}{4} = 1$$

$$\frac{56}{71} \times \frac{71}{56} = 1 \qquad \frac{2}{3} \times \frac{3}{2} = 1$$

Do these problems make *sense*?

DIVISION OF FRACTIONS

To divide a fraction by a whole number, multiply the fraction by the reciprocal of the whole number:

Example 1

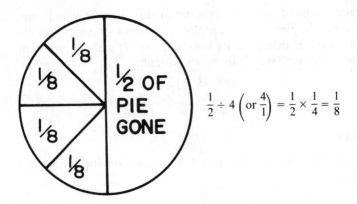

$$\frac{1}{2} \div 4 \left(\text{or } \frac{4}{1} \right) = \frac{1}{2} \times \frac{1}{4} = \frac{1}{8}$$

This problem would answer the following question. If there is 1/2 of a pie left, and 4 people are to get equal pieces, how much of the whole pie will each person get? From the equation above, and the accompanying illustration, it can be seen that each person will get 1/4 of the 1/2 pie, or 1/8 of the whole pie. He will get 1 of 8 equal parts that make up the whole pie; 4/8 or four 1/8-pieces equal 1/2 of the whole pie.

To divide one fraction by another fraction, invert the divisor (turn it upside-down) and multiply:

Example 2

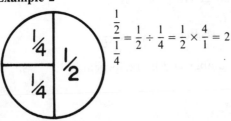

$$\frac{\frac{1}{2}}{\frac{1}{4}} = \frac{1}{2} \div \frac{1}{4} = \frac{1}{2} \times \frac{4}{1} = 2$$

This problem would answer the following question. How many 1/4 pieces of pie are there in 1/2 of a pie? Note that when dividing a fraction (or a whole number) by a fraction, the quotient is *always* larger than the dividend.

DECIMAL FRACTIONS

Since the metric system is used extensively in problems of drugs and solutions, learning to work with decimal fractions is extremely important. The metric system is a decimal system of weights and measures. A decimal fraction is a fraction whose denominator is 10, or any power of 10, i.e., 100, 1,000, 10,000, etc. The denominator, however, is not written as it is in a common fraction. It is signified by the way the number to the right of a decimal point is written.

Example

The fraction 1/2 is easily converted to a decimal fraction by dividing the numerator by the denominator, thus:

$$\frac{1}{2} = 2\overline{\smash{)}1.0}^{\;.5}$$

$$\frac{1 \text{ (numerator)}}{2 \text{ (denominator)}} = .5 \text{ (quotient)}$$

The quotient can also be written 5/10 since $(1 \times 5)/(2 \times 5) = 5/10$; both 5/10 and .5 are read as five-tenths.

Metric Scale

Whole numbers are written to the left of a decimal point. Fractions are written to the right of a decimal point.

Billions	Hundred-millions	Ten-millions	Millions	Hundred-thousands	Ten-thousands	Thousands	Hundreds	Tens	Units	Decimal point	Tenths	Hundredths	Thousandths	Ten-thousandths	Hundred-thousandths	Millionths	Ten-millionths	Hundred-millionths	Billionths	Ten-billionths
10	9	8	7	6	5	4	3	2	1	.	1	2	3	4	5	6	7	8	9	10

Examples

The number 54,321.12345 is read: fifty-four thousand, three hundred twenty-one *and* twelve thousand three hundred forty-five hundred-thousandths.

The number 310.0546 is read: three hundred ten *and* five hundred forty-six ten-thousandths.

The word "and" signifies the decimal point, and is the only way in which the word "and" can be used correctly in expressing a number. In reading numbers, "and" *always* means the decimal point.

Addition and Subtraction of Decimal Fractions

When adding or subtracting decimal fractions, the decimal points must be directly under each other. Add as many zeros after the decimal point as are needed.

Example 1: Add 2.5 + .065 + 25.75 + 2075.009

2.5	two *and* five-tenths
.065	sixty-five thousandths
25.75	twenty-five *and* seventy-five hundredths
+2075.009	two thousand seventy-five *and* nine thousandths
sum 2103.324	two thousand one hundred three *and* three hundred twenty-four thousandths

Example 2: Subtract 26.0076 from 34.1

34.1000	thirty-four *and* one-tenth (add 3 zeros for necessary subtraction)
−26.0076	twenty-six *and* seventy-six ten-thousandths
remainder 8.0924	eight *and* nine hundred twenty-four ten-thousandths

Multiplication of Decimal Fractions

To multiply decimal fractions, the math is the same as with whole numbers. After the product has been figured, count the number of decimal places in *both* the multiplier and the multiplicand. Then, starting from the right of the product, count off this total number of decimal places toward the left, and place the decimal point there.

Example 3: Multiply 24.2 by 6.4

```
    24.2  multiplicand
     6.4  multiplier
    9 68
   145 2
   154.88 product
```

Count the places to the right of the decimal point in the multiplier: 6.4 has 1 place to the right of the decimal point. Count the places to the right of the decimal point in the multiplicand: 24.2 has 1 place to the right of the decimal point. Add the places just counted: $1 + 1 = 2$ decimal places. Counting off 2 places from right to left, the decimal point is placed as is shown above, in the product.

Example 4: Multiply 24.00065 × .002

```
   24.00065  multiplicand
 ×     .002  multiplier
  .04800130  product
```

Count the places to the right of the decimal point in the multiplier:

.002 has 3 decimal places. Count the places to the right of the decimal point in the multiplicand: 24.00065 has 5 decimal places. Add the decimal places just counted: $3 + 5 = 8$ decimal places. Counting off 8 places from right to left, we see that the product, 4800130 has only 7 places. Since the product has fewer places than the required number of places, a zero is added to the left of the last number in the product as shown above. The product is:

$$.0\ 4\ 8\ 0\ 0\ 1\ 3\ \emptyset$$

$$(\ 8\ 7\ 6\ 5\ 4\ 3\ 2\ 1 \leftarrow counting)$$

Do these answers make *sense*?

Division of Decimal Fractions

To divide decimal fractions, the math is the same as with whole numbers. If there are no decimal places in the divisor, place the decimal point in the quotient directly above the decimal point in the dividend.

Example 1: Divide 15.75 by 75

```
                      .21  quotient
       Divisor   75 )15.75  dividend
                    15 0
                    ─────
                      75
                      75
                    ─────
```

If there are decimals in the divisor only, place a decimal point after the whole number of the dividend. Make the divisor a whole number by moving the decimal point to the right of the number. Count off the same number of decimal places in the dividend in the same direction as in the divisor, i.e., to the right, adding zeros, as necessary. Place the decimal point in the quotient directly above this new decimal point in the dividend.

Example 2: Divide 30 by 1.436

$$1.436\ )\overline{30.}$$

Place a decimal point after the 30. Move the decimal point to the right in the divisor until it is a whole number; 1.436 becomes 1436. The decimal point has been moved 3 places to the right. Move the decimal point in the dividend the same number of places as it was moved in the divisor, adding a zero at each place; 30 becomes 30000. The problem now looks like this:

$$1436\ )\overline{30000.}$$

The decimal point in the quotient has been placed directly above the new decimal point in the dividend. The division is done exactly as it is for whole numbers:

$$\frac{20.891 + \text{remainder}}{1436 \overline{)30000.000}}$$

If both the dividend and the divisor contains decimals, make the divisor a whole number, as above, and move the decimal point in the dividend the same number of decimal places to the right as it was moved in the divisor. Then put the decimal point in the quotient directly above the new decimal point in the dividend.

Example 3: Divide .04284 by .68

$$.68 \overline{).04284} \quad \text{becomes} \quad 68 \overline{)4.284}^{\,.063}$$

As is true in dividing a common fraction by another common fraction, the quotient found from dividing a decimal fraction by another decimal fraction is *always greater* than the dividend.

Do these answers make *sense*?

MULTIPLYING AND DIVIDING DECIMAL FRACTIONS BY POWERS OF 10

It was stated earlier that a decimal fraction is a fraction whose denominator is 10, or any power of 10, i.e., 100, 1,000, 10,000, 100,000, etc. and is expressed by the number written to the right of the decimal point. A very easy way to multiply decimal fractions by 10 is to move the decimal point 1 place to the right; to multiply by 100, move the decimal point 2 places to the right, and so forth.

Example 1

$$.4 \times 10 = 4.0$$
$$.4 \times 100 = 40.0$$
$$.4 \times 1,000 = 400.0$$
$$.4 \times 10,000 = 4,000.0$$

To multiply by powers of 10, move the decimal point 1 place to the right for each 0 in the multiplier.

To divide decimal fractions by 10, move the decimal point to the left 1 place; to divide by 100, move the decimal point 2 places to the left. To divide by powers of 10, move the decimal point to the left 1 place for each 0 in the divisor.

Example 2

$$4,000 \div 10 = 400.0$$
$$4,000 \div 100 = 40.00$$
$$4,000 \div 1,000 = 4.000$$
$$4,000 \div 10,000 = .4000$$

EXPONENTS OF 10

Powers of 10 are often expressed by exponents. A positive exponent signifies a whole number:

Examples

$$100 = 10^2$$
$$1,000 = 10^3$$
$$10,000 = 10^4$$
$$100,000 = 10^5$$

A negative exponent signifies a decimal fraction:

$$.1 = 10^{-1} = 1/10$$
$$.01 = 10^{-2} = 1/10^2 = 1/100$$
$$.001 = 10^{-3} = 1/10^3 = 1/1,000$$
$$.0001 = 10^{-4} = 1/10^4 = 1/10,000$$

The shorthand method for expressing astronomical numbers is by the use of exponents of 10. A positive exponent after the number 10 indicates the number of places to move the decimal point to the right, adding zeros, as necessary:

Example 1

$$109. \times 10^4 = 109. \times 10 \times 10 \times 10 \times 10 = 1,090,000.$$

Each place added to the right multiplies the number by 10.

Example 2

$$6.02 \times 10^{23} \doteq 602,000,000,000,000,000,000,000$$

A negative exponent after the number 10 indicates the number of places to move the decimal point to the left, adding zeros, as necessary:

Example 1

$$109. \times 10^{-4} = 109. \div 10 \div 10 \div 10 \div 10 = .0109$$

Each place that the decimal point is moved to the left divides the number by 10.

Example 2

$$40 \times 10^{-9} = .000\ 000\ 04\emptyset$$

This number has the same value as 4×10^{-8}, or .000 000 04.

Exponent Method of Adding and Subtracting by Powers of 10

Example 1: Add $(3.56 \times 10^9) + (607.2 \times 10^5)$

The long method: Change the numbers so that they have no exponents:

$$
\begin{array}{r}
3{,}560{,}000{,}000 \\
+\quad 60{,}720{,}000 \\
\hline
3{,}620{,}720{,}000 = 3.62072 \times 10^9
\end{array}
$$

The exponent method: Change the exponents of the addends so that they are the same; place the decimal points directly under each other; and add:

$$607.2 \times 10^5 = .06072 \times 10^9$$

$$
\begin{array}{r}
3.56\quad \times 10^9 \\
+\ .06072 \times 10^9 \\
\hline
3.62072 \times 10^9 = 3{,}620{,}720{,}000
\end{array}
$$

Notice that the exponents of 10 remain the same. The answers are the same using both methods.

Example 2: Subtract 607×10^3 from 105.4×10^4

The long method: Change the numbers so that they have no exponents, and subtract:

$$
\begin{array}{r}
1054000 \\
-\ 607000 \\
\hline
447000 = 44.7 \times 10^4
\end{array}
$$

The exponent method: Change the exponents of the minuend and the subtrahend so that they are the same. Place the decimal points directly under each other, and subtract:

$$607 \times 10^3 = 60.7 \times 10^4$$

$$
\begin{array}{r}
105.4 \times 10^4 \\
-\ 60.7 \times 10^4 \\
\hline
44.7 \times 10^4 = 447000
\end{array}
$$

Notice that the exponents of 10 remain the same. The remainders are the same using both methods.

Exponent Method of Multiplying by Powers of 10

Example 1: Multiply $(105 \times 10^4) \times (607 \times 10^3)$

The long method:

$$
\begin{array}{r}
1050000 \\
\times \quad 607000 \\
\hline
637{,}350{,}000{,}000 = 63{,}735 \times 10^7
\end{array}
$$

The exponent method: To multiply by exponents of 10, add the exponent of the multiplicand to the exponent of the multiplier.

$$
\begin{array}{r}
105 \times 10^4 \\
\times \quad 607 \times 10^3 \\
\hline
63{,}735 \times 10^7
\end{array}
$$

Step 1 Multiply the numbers involved in the conventional way.
Step 2 Add the exponents of the multiplicand and the multiplier.
Step 3 Combine the answers obtained in steps 1 and 2.

Notice that this answer is identical to the answer found by multiplying in the conventional, long method.

Example 2: Multiply

$$
\begin{array}{r}
6.02 \times 10^{23} \\
\times \quad 4. \times 10^{-8} \\
\hline
24.08 \times 10^{15} = 24{,}080{,}000{,}000{,}000{,}000
\end{array}
$$

The exponents in this example are added thus:

$$23 + (-8) =$$
$$23 - 8 = +15$$

Exponent Method of Dividing by Powers of 10

Example 1: Divide

$$(10496 \times 10^8) \div (309 \times 10^4)$$

The long method:

$$
\begin{array}{r}
\cdot 339676. + \text{remainder} \\
3090000\,\overline{)1049600000000}
\end{array}
$$

The exponent method: To divide by exponents of 10, subtract the exponent of the divisor from the exponent of the dividend.
Step 1 Divide

$$
\begin{array}{r}
33.9676 + \\
309\,\overline{)10496.0000}
\end{array}
$$

Step 2   Subtract the exponent of the divisor from the exponent of the dividend.

$$\begin{array}{r} 10^8 \\ -10^4 \\ \hline 10^4 \end{array}$$

Step 3   Combine the answers found in steps 1 and 2.

$$33.9676+ \times 10^4 = 339,676. + \text{remainder}$$

Notice that this answer is identical to the answer found by dividing in the long method.

Example 2: Divide

$$(1 \times 10^{-14}) \div (1 \times 10^{-2}) = 1 \times 10^{-12}$$

Subtract the exponent of the divisor from the exponent of the dividend.

$$(-14) - (-2) = -14 + 2 = -12$$

Example 3: Divide

$$(1 \times 10^{-14}) \div (4 \times 10^{-8})$$

Step 1   Divide the numbers involved.

$$4 \overline{\smash{)}1.00} \quad .25$$

Step 2   Subtract the exponent of the divisor from the exponent of the dividend.

$$\frac{10^{-14}}{10^{-8}} = 10^{-6}$$

$$-14 - (-8) = -14 + 8 = -6$$

Step 3   Combine the answers obtained in steps 1 and 2.

$$.25 \times 10^{-6} \text{ or } .00000025$$

$$(1 \times 10^{-14}) \div (4 \times 10^{-8}) = .25 \times 10^{-6}$$

This review should prepare the student for mastering the material in this text. If exceptional weakness is apparent after this review, it is suggested that before proceeding further, the student seek other elementary texts on the subject, and practice with many problems until he feels competent to use these mathematical calculations.

Bibliography

1. Downie, N. M., and Heath, R. W. 1965. *Basic Statistical Methods,* 2nd Ed. New York: Harper and Row.
2. Egan, D. F. 1969. *Fundamentals of Inhalation Therapy,* St. Louis: Mosby.
3. Freund, J. E. 1960. *Modern Elementary Statistics,* 2nd ed., Englewood Cliffs, N.J.: Prentice-Hall.
4. Goodman, L. S., and Gilman, A. 1970. *The Pharmacological Basis of Therapeutics,* 4th ed. New York: MacMillan.
5. Guyton, A. C. 1971. *Basic Human Physiology,* Philadelphia: Saunders.
6. Guyton, A. C. 1971. *Textbook of Medical Physiology,* 4th ed. Philadelphia: Saunders.
7. Huff, D. 1954. *How to Lie with Statistics,* New York: Norton.
8. Morris, W., ed. 1969. *American Heritage Dictionary of the English Language,* New York: Houghton Mifflin.
9. Shapiro, B. A. 1977. *Clinical Applications of Blood Gases,* 2nd ed. Chicago: Year Book Medical.
10. Smith, R. M. 1968. *Anesthesia for Infants and Children,* 3rd ed. St. Louis: Mosby.
11. Wilson, C. O. 1971. *Textbook of Organic, Medicinal, and Pharmaceutical Chemistry,* 6th ed. Philadelphia: Lippincott.
12. Wylie, W. D., Churchill-Davidson, H. C. 1972. *A Practice of Anesthesia,* 3rd ed. Chicago: Year Book Medical.

INDEX